Understanding Substance Use

Critical Approaches to Social Work

Other books you may be interested in:

Anti-Racism in Social Work Practice
Edited by Angie Bartoli
ISBN 978-1-909330-13-9

Modern Mental Health: Critical Perspectives on Psychiatric Practice
Edited by Steven Walker
ISBN 978-1-909330-53-5

Positive Social Work: The Essential Toolkit for NQSWs
By Julie Adams and Angie Sheard
ISBN 978-1-909330-05-4

Evidencing CPD – A Guide to Building Your Social Work Portfolio
By Daisy Bogg and Maggie Challis
ISBN 978-1-909330-25-2

Personal Safety for Social Workers and Health Professionals
By Brian Atkins
ISBN 978-1-909330-33-7

What's Your Problem? Making Sense of Social Policy and the Policy Process
By Stuart Connor
ISBN 978-1-909330-49-8

Starting Social Work – Reflections of a Newly Qualified Social Worker
By Rebecca Joy Novell
ISBN 978-1-909682-09-2

Titles are also available in a range of electronic formats. To order please go to our website www.criticalpublishing.com or contact our distributor NBN International, 10 Thornbury Road, Plymouth PL6 7PP, telephone 01752 202301 or email orders@nbninternational.com

Understanding Substance Use
Policy and Practice

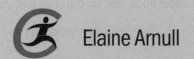

Elaine Arnull

Critical Approaches to Social Work

First published in 2014 by Critical Publishing Ltd.

British Library Cataloguing in Publication Data
A CIP record for this book is available from the British Library

ISBN: 978-1-909330-93-1

This book is also available in the following e-book formats:

Kindle ISBN: 978-1-909330-94-8
EPUB ISBN: 978-1-909330-95-5
Adobe e-book ISBN: 978-1-909330-96-2

Cover design by Greensplash Limited
Project Management by Out of House Publishing
Typeset by Newgen KnowledgeWorks Pvt Ltd, India
Printed and bound in Great Britain by Bell and Bain, Glasgow

Critical Publishing
152 Chester Road
Northwich
CW8 4AL
www.criticalpublishing.com

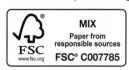

Contents

Acknowledgements

I would like to thank many people for their help and support with this book. I am grateful to two people who read chapters of the book and advised me to ensure my perspective was balanced and up to date; they are my colleague Jane Wright, Senior Lecturer Bucks New University and Colin MacGregor, Chief Executive Oasis, Drug Treatment Provider, Bucks and Oxon. Any errors or omissions are my own.

I would also like to thank my husband Conor and my daughter Morgan for their immense support through everything and their acceptance of the disruptions caused to our family life that writing seems to bring. Thank you too to my mother Pat who has always supported my educational efforts and helps to publicise my books.

Finally, I would like to thank Di who has been a supportive and constructive Editor and who has driven the process forward and cared deeply about the quality of the outcome.

Meet the author

Elaine's research has attracted international attention and exerted an influence on policy and practice. Her principle focus has been on social policy and in particular the effect of policy in the area of substance use and the policy and practice area of young people, offending and juvenile justice. She has published widely in these areas and undertaken large-scale, innovative research.

Elaine is a qualified social worker and worked for a number of years as a Probation Officer. Since 1999 she has researched, taught and worked in Higher Education; she is interested in developing thinking and practice concerned with the interface between theory, research, social policy and practice. She serves on a number of Boards aimed at further developing thinking and work in this area.

Acronyms

AA	Alcoholics Anonymous
ACMD	Advisory Council on the Misuse of Drugs
ACPO	Association of Chief Police Officers
ADAT	Alcohol and Drug Action Team
A&E	Accident and Emergency
AOP	Anti-Oppressive Practice
ASBO	Anti-Social Behaviour Order
BASW	British Association of Social Work
BCS	British Crime Survey
BME	Black and Minority Ethnic
CARAT	Counselling – Advice – Referral – Assessment – Throughcare (team)
CBT	Cognitive Behavioural Therapy
CDCU	Central Drugs Coordination Unit
CDRP	Crime and Disorder Reduction Partnership
CEO	Chief Executive (Officer)
CJIP	Community Justice Intervention Programme
CJIT	Community Justice Intervention Team
CJS	Criminal Justice System
CSEW	Crime Survey of England and Wales
CSR	Comprehensive Spending Review
CTDM	Crack Treatment Delivery Model
DAAT	Drug and Alcohol Action Team
DAMS	Drug and Alcohol Monitoring System
DAT	Drug Action Team
DCSF	Department for Children, Schools and Families
DDAC	District Drug Advisory Committee
DoH	Department of Health
DIP	Drug Intervention Programme
DIR	Drug Interventions Record
DPAS	Drug Prevention Advisory Service
DPI	Drug Prevention Initiative
DRG	Drug Reference Group
DRR	Drug Rehabilitation Requirement
DSD	Drug Strategy Directorate
DTTO	Drug Treatment and Testing Order

EAZ	Education Action Zone
EMCDDA	European Monitoring Centre on Drugs and Drug Addiction
GO	Government Office
HA	Health Authority
HAZ	Health Action Zone
HCPC	Health and Care Professions Council
HO	Home Office
IDTS	Integrated Drug Treatment System
ISDD	Institute for the Study of Drug Dependence
IV	Intravenous (drug use)
KPI	Key Performance Indicator
LA	Local Authorities
LHB	Local Health Board
Localities	used to denote the local area and/or DAT, as opposed to the 'centre'
LSP	Local Strategic Partnership
MASH	Multi-Agency Safeguarding Hub
MI	Motivational Interviewing
MP	Member of Parliament
NA	Narcotics Anonymous
NCA	National Crime Agency
NHS	National Health Service
NICE	National Institute for Health and Care Excellence
NPM	New Performance Management
NPS	New Psychoactive Substance
NTA	National Treatment Agency
NTORS	National Treatment Outcome Research Study
OAS	Organization of American States
ODPM	Office of the Deputy Prime Minister
PbR	Payment by Results
PCT	Primary Care Trust
PHE	Public Health England
PM	Prime Minister
RCT	Randomised Control Trial
RDMD	Regional Drug Misuse Database
SCODA	Standing Conference on Drug Abuse
SEU	Social Exclusion Unit
SIB	Social Impact Bond
SLA	Service Level Agreement
SRA	Social Research Association
TDT	Tackling Drugs Together
TDTBBB	Tackling Drugs to Build a Better Britain
UKADCU	UK Anti-Drugs Coordination Unit
UKDPC	UK Drug Policy Commission
VFM	Value For Money
YJS	Youth Justice System
YOTs	Youth Offending Teams

Summary of initiatives

During the period covered in this book there have been numerous new policies, reports and initiatives, some of which were quickly superseded and others which remained in force. Some of the key policies and initiatives introduced during this period (or preceding it but of relevance) are shown chronologically in the table below; this list is by no means exhaustive. The range of policies and initiatives also helps to give a flavour of how deeply embedded in all forms of government activity drug and latterly alcohol policy has become.

1928   International Convention for Narcotics Control
1961   Single Convention on Narcotic Drugs
1971   Convention on Psychotropic Substances
1984   Social Services Committee Report
1985   Cabinet Ministerial Sub-Committee on Drugs Misuse created
1988   Convention against Illicit Traffic in Narcotic Drugs and Psychotropic Substances (1988)
1995   Tackling Drugs Together – White Paper
1996   The Task Force to Review Services for Drug Misusers
1998   Tackling Drugs to Build a Better Britain
        Modern Public Services for Britain: Investing in Reform: Comprehensive Spending Review Plans 1999–2002
        Crime and Disorder Act (lays provision for Drug Treatment and Testing Orders – DTTOs)
1999   Modernising Government (Cmd 4310)
2000   Police Foundation Report
        Criminal Justice and Court Services Act (creates Drug Abstinence Order – DAO)
2001   Proceeds of Crime Bill (CM5066)
        Communities Against Drugs (CAD) fund
2002   Updated Drug Strategy
        Models of care for the treatment of drug misusers (national framework for commissioning substance misuse services)
        National Crack Action Plan
        Proceeds of Crime Bill
        Police Reform Act
        Home Affairs Committee Report: The Government's Drug Policy: Is it Working? (HC318)

2003   Criminal Justice Act (replaces DTTO with Drug Rehabilitation Requirement – DRR)
        Criminal Justice Intervention Project (CJIP – later becomes known as Drugs
        Intervention Programme – DIP)
        Building Safer Communities Fund (BSCF – changed from CAD)
        FRANK drug information campaign
        Licensing Act
        Police Reform Act
2004   Tackling drugs: changing lives: delivering the difference
        Tackling drugs: changing lives. Every child matters: change for children: young
        people and drugs
        Tackling drugs – changing lives. Keeping communities safe from drugs
2005   Tackling drugs – changing lives. Turning strategy into reality
        The Drugs Act
2006   Select Committee on Science and Technology Fifth Report (CM200506)
2007   Drugs, Our Community, Your Say
2008   Drugs: Protecting Families and Communities
2010   Drug Strategy
2011   Police Reform Act
        Police Reform and Social Responsibility Act 2011
2012   Alcohol Strategy 2012
2013   National Crime Agency
        Public Health England – replaced NTA responsibilities for drug use

incidence of blood-borne disease and drug-related deaths, but you might also see interviews with the IV drug users to ascertain how accessible was the service, etc. Therefore when reading research in this area (as in general) ask yourself, do the methods chosen enable the question to be answered?

There are numerous studies of prevalence of drug use in particular in the UK and most of these post-date the first drug strategy, TDT 1995, thus data usually relate to the recent past. There was a real issue in the late 1980s and early 1990s about understanding how widespread the problem of drug use was. As we have discussed, drug issues and treatment were largely a 'Cinderella' area in health in the early 1990s, and those who were concerned about what they saw as a changing pattern of drug use with criminal justice impacts felt they had little opportunity to understand or investigate it. The effect of these tensions was real and it was not a purely academic or scientific debate: for example if one does not know what is being used, how much, by whom, when and under what circumstances with any level of certainty, you cannot plan for services, treatment or anticipate impacts. An indication of what this meant, and the tensions around in relation was given by one Mott who, speaking from a Home Office research perspective describing the 1970s and 1980s,

> remember, whoever counted could be an 'accountant', so there was question
> of epidemiology, it all seemed to centre on the 'tip' of a iceberg and it ended up with
> problems, I was putting questions in, trying to help, even to the British Crime Survey.
>
> (Mott 2000: 289)

Thus, tensions and debates about who had the right to deal with drugs issues and how those varying perspectives could be debated, integrated and brought together, had a direct impact on policy, service delivery, law and the ability to 'know' what was happening through research. These were the days before 'joined-up' government, and they serve as a reminder of the very discrete ways in which the big institutions of state operated. Moreover, the introduction of the questions on the British Crime Survey (BCS) turned out to be very useful regarding the question of drug trying and its wider impacts and these have continued although they have become more sophisticated over time. The survey has now changed its name to become the Crime Survey of England and Wales (CSEW).

Organisations such as the DATs, DH, DPAS and later the NTA, in response to the various government strategies, have since the mid 1990s also increased the amount that we now know about drug use, drug trying and other health, criminal justice and social effects. Finally Europe also now features the collection and collation of large amounts of epidemiological data and commissions other types of research, including in depth qualitative studies.

The interesting thing about substance use is that it is an ever-changing scene and therefore this book will concentrate on ensuring an understanding of how and of going issues and debates, as well as presenting some headline figures and issues with which policy makers are currently grappling. Once again the best place to follow in detail the current patterns of use and supply is through the government and EMCDDA websites.

The EMCDDA (2012a) report highlights concerns about the impact of the economic and financial downturn in Europe and its potential to impact drug use. It suggests that countries need to think clearly about the costs and benefits of drug treatment services and identifies six countries in Europe that have made recent cuts to specified drug budgets; these include

1 Introduction

Drugs and alcohol are hotly debated features of our society. They have been a focus for discussion throughout history and moral arguments and judgements have formed recurring themes in that discourse.

This book addresses the areas of substance use policy and practice; it considers changes to drug and alcohol policy that have occurred since the first drug policy, Tackling Drugs Together in 1995. The policy changes incorporated into that policy have formed the basic architecture that subsequent policies have incorporated; this includes an emphasis on partnership at a policy and practice level. Directions during this period have included debates and discussion about community and respect, about individual vs collective rights, about libertarian freedoms and the role of the criminal justice system. The trajectory of policy and the debate that surrounds it do therefore mirror those within the wider social policy arena, although the moral attributes or deficits ascribed to those who use substances or work within the treatment sphere may be more keenly ascribed than in other areas.

The pace of change for social policy has been fast since the late 1990s and for drug and alcohol policy this has been acute – many of those involved have expressed and continue to express an inability to 'keep up' with the changes to policy, delivery and rhetoric. For students from a variety of backgrounds interested in the area or intending to work or practice within a field touched by substance use this scale and pace of change can make the area seem overwhelming and the area unknowable. And yet few people's lives in the UK or much of the developed world will be untouched by substance use, either within their personal or family life, within their world of work, their social sphere or the media they consume. Making this connection between the personal and the learning and working environment may seem uncomfortable and some will argue irrelevant. However, because substance use touches the lives of most, it provokes deep-seated feelings, reactions and values which may be unrecognised; learning in this area and perhaps practising in this area requires a recognition of that personal orientation and this book consistently asks the reader to consider and make those connections. This area of social policy is heavily value laden and it affects all aspects of policy-making, practice delivery and the discussion and debate which then surround them. This can be seen in the terms that are chosen by the discussant, for example 'use', 'dependence' or 'addiction'. It influences the way in which famous people talk about their own substance use and the way the media reports on or portrays that. It informs the way individuals, organisations and communities respond to health prevention programmes such as the debate recently surrounding unit pricing of alcohol and the provision of safe injecting rooms in Brighton, England. If policy is to be made that is based on conceptions of minimising harm, and practice is anti-oppressive then it is incumbent upon those working in those spheres, researching them, analysing, informing and commenting on them to be quite clear about whence their reactions, attitudes and values come and to be quite explicit how that informs and shapes their responses; this book through its discussion and representation of policy and practice within the arena of substance use seeks to engage the reader in that debate and journey.

Current policy and practice in the UK regarding substance use is moving towards a model of localism and away from central direction and advice. Service provision is increasingly influenced by market philosophies such as payment by results (PbR) and impacted by the deep cuts to public services budgets in general, for example the UK is one of those noted by the European Monitoring Centre on Drugs and Drug Addiction (EMCDDA 2012c), as having some of the biggest recent budget cuts to drug policy and provision within Europe. Prior to this in recent years the approach had been towards a heavy investment in services and provision, some of which were accessed via the criminal justice system. Current philosophies within the policy and practice spheres talk of a recovery model, recognising the many attempts that may be taken towards controlling drug and alcohol use or living free from dependence. While the discourse is valuable because it recognises the journey someone may make and the range of services they may need to access over many years of their life in order to make the changes they may wish to make, it appears at odds with the powerful discourse about reducing the state, budget cuts and PbR, to be incongruent with recent government responses which have been to ignore expert advice regarding harm, cannabis and khat classifications and the apparently increasingly moralised and judgemental approach to alcohol use; as ever therefore, substance use policy provides an interesting microcosm for all sorts of wider structural, social and policy debates.

The partnership framework for policy and practice delivery regarding substance use has been strengthened by the current moves towards a recovery agenda and it will be interesting to see how this takes effect in the forthcoming period. As noted there is considerable tension both philosophically and in practice with other policy moves towards PbR initiatives and budget cuts and at this stage it is unknown how these cuts will impact and which groups will be considered most deserving of tax payers' money. The partnership style of working and the different routes by which treatment can be accessed mean that a wide variety of professional groups work with drug and alcohol users and need to acquire a generic, but educated understanding of substance use policy and practice and the debates within and surrounding it; the group who require in-depth specialist skills and knowledge are much smaller. The need for generic professionals to become more knowledgeable about substance use is considered to be acute and this book considers the evidence in this area in some depth.

The book considers the creation and formation of drug and alcohol policy up to the present period (2013) and then considers how this has shaped practice and treatment approaches and how in turn all have been impacted by wider structural, social, cultural and international forces. Substance use policy is contexualised within the UK and a wider global setting in order for the scale of the issue to be properly understood. The latter chapters discuss treatment and practice approaches, and the language and assumptions that surround and drive them. National and international research informs each chapter and the reader is guided towards original and more specialist, in-depth sources where they might wish to know more or follow up on a particular context. Throughout the book there is a focus on understanding oneself and ensuring that as a reader, consumer, commentator, policy maker, researcher or practitioner you are self-aware, non-judgemental and not oppressive towards others in the comments you make or the actions you take. As you will see, how you might achieve this within this area is not always clear and may in itself be hotly contested; it is always what makes this area exciting, challenging and constantly changing.

Overview of the chapters

Chapter 2 considers the UK's first drug policy, Tackling Drugs Together (TDT) (1995), and why it emerged. It reflects upon why partnership work became integral to work within the substance use field and how this affected and shaped it. In addition, the chapter briefly considers how ideas that emerged from the drug policies affected the ways in which drug and alcohol use and users were viewed in the years that followed. Thus, the moralisation of drug use and users during this period and how this was aligned with notions of community is discussed in some depth.

TDT is discussed in some detail because the architecture and overarching principles have remained intact and been carried forward into subsequent policies. Understanding how and why those were constructed as they were is critical to developing an understanding of subsequent and current policy and the trajectory that now affects and informs the responses to alcohol use. It also introduces key concepts such as harm minimisation, which has continued to be controversial in policy terms but effective as a practice response.

Chapter 3 builds on Chapter 2, focusing on drug and then alcohol policy post-1998. It looks at how the wider social policy analysis taken by New Labour and applied to drugs policy affected and shaped their strategies. We also look at recurring themes such as the moralisation of substance use and concerns about harm minimisation approaches and consider whether or not high levels of central focus, considerable amounts of money and an alignment with a crime agenda affected the policy directions and outcomes. Finally we look at subsequent drug and alcohol policy including the increasingly emergent and urgent nature of the latter. We also consider apparent changes in focus such as PbR, a loss of central direction and a move towards what is argued to be a 'recovery'-based agenda.

Chapter 4 focuses on the social and legal context of substance use and how this is shaped by cultural, social and historical factors including, for example, geography. A brief description of the Misuse of Drugs Act 1971 and the 1998 Crime and Disorder Act and other relevant legislation is included, and the reader is pointed to more specialist texts. The chapter sites legal restrictions within the context of other analyses of the 'harms' related to substance use that are advanced by academics such as Professor David Nutt (2010) and campaign groups such the UK Drug Policy Commission (UKDPC 2012) and those arguing for legalisation such as Transform. This includes a discussion of the policy directions and debate in the wider international policy world regarding legalisation, decriminalisation and policy 'experiments' in Switzerland and Portugal, and moves within the Organization of American States (OAS) to change policy focus. The reader is thereby enabled to engage with substance use policy as something that has a national cultural context as well as international implications, responsibilities and ramifications.

The chapter explores further how legal constructs affect the moral view of substance use and users and considers how substance users can be created as the 'other' and how this can be harmful to good practice and effective engagement; this contention is further explored from an anti-oppressive practice (AOP) perspective. This is also discussed within its international context.

Chapter 5 considers why people think substance use is a problem and draws on epidemiological studies regarding prevalence to understand more about the scale of the issue. Research findings are explored in order to elucidate the impact of substance use on particular groups – for example children and young people, women, black and minority ethnic (BME) groups, older people, and in relation to mental health and terms such as 'dual diagnosis'. An anti-oppressive framework is used to allow the reader to consider how difficult it can be for different groups of service users and their families and friends to discuss or report the effects or scope of substance use and how effective engagement can help to overcome these concerns.

Chapter 6 presents the dominant treatment and intervention approaches to substance misuse which includes a discussion of the concepts of harm reduction, dependency and addiction and their impact on treatment approaches. It also includes consideration of the recent move in treatment and commissioning approaches away from 'tiers' and towards 'layers' of treatment (Strang 2012). What both 'tiers' and 'layers' attempt to describe is the type and range of interventions that can be found, the sorts of practitioners who would be involved at each stage and the type and depth of knowledge they would need; a table is included to help the reader visualise what this looks like in practice.

Chapters 4, 5 and 6 are therefore more explicitly orientated towards consideration of the impact of practice relevant to the arenas of social work, social care, the criminal justice system (CJS) and youth justice system (YJS), psychological services and healthcare, such as health visitors, school and district nurses. They should be read in conjunction with Chapters 2 and 3, which set the context for how to then interpret and understand the policy context within which practice is framed. All are relevant for those researching or working in policy and wanting to understand more about the interface between policy and practice.

The final chapter, 7, is principally focused on a series of exercises, which enable the reader independently (or a lecturer/teacher/trainer to explore with a class or group) the issues raised within the book. The exercises can be undertaken independently or sequentially and help to further explore key issues; they are explicitly orientated towards engaging with the policy and practice issues surrounding substance use in a way that is reflective. The intention is to enable and encourage critical, reflective thinking, which aids deep learning (Arnull and Aldridge-Bent 2013).

2 Social policy: the first strategy – Tackling Drugs Together

Introduction

This chapter will address key issues: What was the nature of the first drug policy in the UK? How and why did it emerge? Why did partnership work become integral and how has this affected the nature of the work? The chapter will later explore how the importance placed on multi-agency working has subsequently shaped both policy and practice.

In addition, the chapter briefly considers how ideas that emerged from the drug policies affected the ways in which we view drug and alcohol use and users. The moralisation of drug use and users is identified alongside notions of community that influenced and informed this reasoning. Moralised conceptions can negatively influence policy and practice and in so doing be harmful to good practice and effective engagement; they are picked up further in the following chapter where we will consider subsequent drug and alcohol policies.

This chapter focuses solely and in some detail on Tackling Drugs Together (1995) because the architecture and overarching principles established in that policy have remained intact and been carried forward in subsequent policies. Understanding how and why those were constructed as they were is therefore critical to developing an understanding of subsequent and current policy and the trajectory that now affects and informs the responses to alcohol use.

The discussion of the policies and their formation in this and the following chapter aims to encourage the reader to adopt a critical approach. It seeks to facilitate an understanding of how policy responses are shaped by history, culture and social factors and thus enable the reader to be able to conceptualise how practice and policy can look very different over time and place; we will consider this further in Chapter 4 and 'the social and legal context of substance use'.

LEARNING OUTCOMES

By the end of this chapter you should be able to:

» Describe the first UK policy on drugs and alcohol.

» Form a critical understanding of the background that helped to shape UK drug and alcohol policy.

» Critically evaluate the key debates on the impact of partnership working in this area.

UK drug and alcohol policy

Drug and alcohol policy in the UK has been formed by a series of policies which have retained the same basic structure and three key areas of focus since the first drug policy in 1995, Tackling Drugs Together.[1] Since then the policies have had similar and recurring features but the emphasis within the policy has changed; the emphasis may be upon policy structure as in the first drugs policy or on links between serious drug use and crime as in later ones.

It is important to understand the historical context and basic features of the first drug policy, TDT (1995), because those features have continued to influence the basic shape of each successive drug policy in England, Wales, Northern Ireland and Scotland. This is particularly so in connection with their features regarding policy implementation, namely multi-agency delivery and in general a multi-party consensus; for this reason the first policy, TDT (1995), is described in much more detail than is subsequently the case for later policies. In addition, the principal arguments that informed the debates about policy formation continue to be features of academic and policy debate (UKDPC 2012). These features include:

* the penal/health divide;

* the relative weight given to target setting and central control as opposed to local flexibility;

* harm minimisation or abstinence models;

* social or medical models, including the influence of biological determinism;

* the relative 'harms' of substances.

Over the years, alcohol policy has come to mirror drug policy much more closely, with similar language, policy structures and concerns about social and 'community' harms coming to the fore. For example the Police Reform and Social Responsibility Act (2011) introduced by the coalition government focused upon the *crime and disorder caused by alcohol and the*

---

[1] TDT 1995 was aimed just at England, but the two New Labour drug policies, Tackling Drugs to Build a Better Britain (1998) and the Updated Strategy (2002) encompassed the UK. The basic architecture of those strategies built on that devised in TDT (1995). The cultural impacts and influences varied within the constituent countries of the UK as they did for regional areas and the urban, suburban and rural areas. The coalition's Alcohol Strategy (2012) is also a UK-wide strategy.

resultant health and social harms. We will discuss and explore this trajectory towards the end of the next chapter.

So in this chapter when we talk of substance use policy we are talking about drug policy and alcohol plays little or no role; as time progresses, however, and we come to current concerns you will see the 'rise' of alcohol and concerns about its use (Chapter 3). As drug use has fallen over this period, problematic alcohol use has increased and the strategies that have been devised to combat this mirror those for drug use; therefore the need to understand how drug policy in the UK was formed is further underlined.

This chapter considers the factors that influenced the development of the strategy, including the differing analyses that emerged from Conservative and Labour MPs about drug misuse. By the time TDT (1995) was launched the differences were subsumed under a broad acceptance that the strategy should be cross-party and cross-departmental, but there is brief consideration of earlier attempts to deal with the drug misuse issue and the areas highlighted by evaluations of those attempts. It is important to look at those historical factors because they influenced TDT (1995) in its final form; these included ensuring that there would be attention from the centre, ie senior ministers and the Prime Minister (PM), and in addition that there would be a clear focus on implementation, ie how the policy would be translated into practice.

The chapter also considers the choice of partnership mechanisms for implementation and why these were a popular choice in the late 1980s and early 1990s; in addition it considers whether they have become a new institution. TDT (1995) was able to be many things to many people; an important factor in a policy seeking to address a difficult social policy area that crossed many departmental boundaries, but was the core business of none. As we shall see, partnership played its role in ensuring this ability to be many things to many people. UKDPC (2012) have subsequently described drug policy as a *wicked issue*:

> *a social problem characterised by resistance to resolution over long periods of time, being fractured by different deeply held values and by being connected to other similarly complex and unresolved issues.*

(UKDPC 2012: 90)

Their typology suggests that the policies of TDT (1995) did not lead to a resolution of drug issues, and that the cross-departmental, cross-political party resolve led neither to easy solutions nor to consistent agreement about how to tackle the issues. It underlines, however, the uniqueness and importance of cross-party agreement and support in 1995 and its continued importance. Being a 'wicked' issue in social policy places substance misuse with other issues that cross 'moral' and political barriers and allegiances, for example: social and health policies concerned with the right of a woman to control her own body and decide on the need for a termination; the right of a person who is terminally ill to choose when and how to die; or in the USA the social and crime control policies that are concerned with the right to bear arms in defence of a constitutional right despite apparent social consequences. These sorts of social policy issues cross party political boundaries and appeal to deeply held views with the opposing sides each calling on moral values and appealing to 'rights' to defend their opposing views. They are often concerned with and juxtapose the rights of the individual and the rights of the community; the ability of individuals to decide for themselves and the ability of the community to influence, or not, those behaviours or decisions. In the UK, partnership and multi-agency working, as well as cross-party agreement, helped to bring into effect a consensus in 1995 to tackle the 'wicked' issue that was drug policy.

The TDT (1995) strategy sought to bring together criminal justice and health agendas to tackle an issue of ever greater social and political concern at a time of deep social and political division. Partnership appears to have been the principal mechanism for uniting these difficult divisions; a mechanism that allowed each area or partner to feel that their needs had been or could be addressed.[2] This form of multi-agency cooperation has subsequently been used with regard to other intractable or 'wicked' issues, for example, youth offending (Fox and Arnull 2013; Arnull 2014). It also forms the basis of a considerable amount of work and innovation around child protection scheduled for 2013 to establish Multi-Agency Safeguarding Hubs (MASH): teams that will involve organisations and different professional groups working together to tackle child abuse at a local level.

Developing drug policy: pre-TDT 1995

The development of drug policy in England and Wales in the early 1990s was characterised by a number of features:

- the changing nature of drug misuse;
- the emergence of HIV/AIDS;
- the strength of cross-party support;
- political factors, such as the Conservative government's poor relationships with local government;
- international developments and relationships, for example strong relationships with the USA and the 'war on drugs';
- the growth of a moral political agenda linked to the collapse of the welfare state and the advent of Thatcherism;
- the development of information management and computer-based systems allowing for increased monitoring and reporting and the growth of 'managerialism';
- the popularity of partnership mechanisms for policy implementation and the development of new forms of governance.

All of these affected and shaped the way the policy was developed and designed for implementation. These issues also impacted the development of drug policy in Scotland and Northern Ireland, although differently for social, cultural and political reasons; drug use in Northern Ireland, for example, has traditionally been lower than in other parts of the UK, for complex multi-faceted political, social and cultural reasons.

---

[2] This and the following chapter draw on original, empirical research on drug policy undertaken towards a PhD by Elaine Arnull. The research was based on a review of key policy documentation and interviews with all key players at the centre involved in forming TDT 1995 and those involved in policy implementation post-TDTBBB 1998; all were guaranteed anonymity. The full reference is shown in the bibliography.

This was a time of exciting social policy change with innovation in many areas, be they multi-agency forms with real power, performance management systems, or harm minimisation – all of which seem unremarkable now, but were then new. The small area of drug policy, owned by no one, with little money, no strong institutional control and thus not very much to lose, gave opportunities for these new ideas to be tried out. TDT (1995) was devised by a group of 'hot house' civil servants some of whom had been 'lent out' to the private sector under a Thatcherite scheme to transform the Civil Service and with them they brought new ideas, a willingness to embrace them and the skills to convince politicians to try them out in a small policy area that belonged to none of the large institutions of state (Arnull 2009).

The concern with drug misuse was shared across the political spectrum and so the need for a policy was largely uncontested. In addition, political cooperation on this issue continued throughout the period despite an emerging difference in attribution of the problem. The PM (John Major) lent his support to the strategy, which was influential with regard to how others might see TDT (1995) and how much emphasis might be placed on its adoption and implementation.

Politicians and other policy actors moved towards a more strategic approach to the 'drug problem' in response to the social imperatives which were emerging in the late 1980s. This led to the creation of a clear policy structure which focused on implementation and which included built-in mechanisms for reporting back to the centre. This new and defined approach sought to be radical and to bring into play some of the emerging social policy agendas of the time – partnership approaches and performance management in particular.

The policy was also one shaped by the emerging central policy concerns with implementation and the ability to evidence this through the use of key performance indicators (KPIs) which would be subsequently monitored. It is important to remember that these were new mechanisms, and organisations in the public and private sector were just getting to grips with the levels of information and control the new technologies could give them. KPIs and central reporting were therefore introduced by a Conservative administration who wanted to clearly demonstrate value for money (VFM); all ideas strongly associated with Thatcherism.

Harm minimisation and HIV/AIDS

Prior to this period, drug misuse had been a rather neglected area. Attention, when given, had settled principally on regulation; thus the 1920 Dangerous Drugs Act, The Brain Report 1965 and the 1971 Misuse of Drugs Act. During the late 1980s and early 1990s this changed and drug policy began to be developed with a new emphasis on combating drug misuse problems as they impacted on society at large.

British responses to drug use, on occasions, had been innovative and were often characterised as different from other European or Atlantic responses. The area of drug misuse was small, highly specialised, quite inward looking and often disparate, peopled by practitioners, organisations and academics who were highly individualistic and not easily directed or controlled. There were a number of instances where changes in practice at a local level drove policy responses that were then accepted and incorporated at a national level. An example of this was 'harm minimisation', developed particularly in response to the transmission of HIV/AIDS infections among intravenous (IV) drug users. Britain later received much international recognition for this policy adoption and the perceived 'control' of the virus within the UK drug-using population,[3] but acceptance was largely driven by a practically focused, governmental need to control public health issues (Berridge 1996: 303). In this sense the policy response to HIV/AIDS and the incorporation of 'harm minimisation' can be seen to epitomise what has often been characterised as the 'British Model', which was a pragmatic and health-focused response to drug use (Stimson 1987; Seddon et al. 2012); it was not therefore driven by a moral imperative.

HIV/AIDS prompted two reports from the Advisory Council on the Misuse of Drugs: one in 1988 (ACMD 1988: 1), which urged action to control against HIV infection and suggested that this was *more pressing or dangerous* than the drugs issue itself, and a subsequent report in 1993 which sought to 'update' the situation and suggested that *greater effort* was *needed to reduce the extent of drug use* (Druglink 1994). The link between the two communities (those with HIV/AIDS and IV drug users) was clear and acknowledged. This led the government to accept (although not necessarily wish to publicise) that the ability of drug misuse to damage the health of the whole population, by the spread of HIV/AIDS from IV drug users through sexual contact with 'non-users', was a threat so great that innovative and radical solutions, such as the provision of injecting equipment to IV drug users, could be contemplated and instituted.[4] It is important to remember that prior to this, harm minimisation as a form of accepted health prevention practice did not exist; health-based assistance to drug users had been principally limited to treatment and prescribed medication, with condoms dispensed by some clinics engaged with sex workers.

Harm minimisation as a policy and practice approach has continued to be sensitive and controversial[5] and in the foreword to *Tackling Drugs Together*, *harm minimisation* (TDT 1995: vii) was acknowledged as one of the four main areas developed during the consultation period. Nonetheless, the White Paper went on to make it clear that any information aimed at minimising harm to drug users *must be coupled with the unambiguous message that abstinence from drugs is the only risk-free option* and thus that *harm reduction should be a means to an end, not an end in itself*.

However, the HIV/AIDS 'threat' can also be seen to signify other changes that were taking place and were less positive. In particular this related to the way in which concerns were generalised beyond drug users per se and increasingly focused on the impact of drug use, or the drug user, on the 'normal' population. HIV/AIDS transmission via drug users showed the potential for substance misuse to 'spill out' from a small and enclosed world and perhaps 'contaminate' the general population (TDT 1995: 23). Current concerns about binge drinking and the social and health effects on otherwise 'law abiding' citizens can be seen to

---

[3] There were differential impacts in cities, for example in Edinburgh, where differences in implementation of this policy led, unfortunately, to differential outcomes for those affected by HIV/AIDS as a result and provided further evidence of its success.

[4] Pearson (1991: 205–7) suggested that the 'abnormally high' HIV prevalence in Edinburgh, Scotland was the result of police activity against harm minimisation policies before the consequences were fully understood; this also seemed to show that the policy had worked elsewhere to control HIV infections in IV drug users.

[5] Recent events have brought the sensitive nature of harm minimisation to the fore again within the arena and in particular within public debate and we will discuss this in later chapters.

have provoked similar concerns. In this way, fears about HIV/AIDS and drug misuse have had an impact beyond the immediate health concerns; the one acknowledged most frequently through the introduction of harm minimisation policies and the other through more widespread concerns about the impact of substance use on the general population.

Changes in drug use and a shared government agenda

The debates about drug misuse in the House of Commons in the late 1980s and early 1990s show an increasing concern with drug misuse issues. In 1984 a Home Affairs Committee report led to the creation of a ministerial group concerned with the misuse of drugs.[6] The characteristics of this group showed what were to become core foundations for the implementation of all subsequent strategies, crucially spanning a variety of government departments with the aim of 'supervising' and 'coordinating' the strategy. The group included the Home Office (HO), Departments of Environment, Education and Health, Scottish and Welsh Offices, Defence and the Paymaster General and Solicitor General. This broad sweep of departments established the cooperative nature of tackling substance misuse issues in the UK through the use of cross-departmental structures and cross-party support; it allowed responsibility to be spread out and support and funds accessed to tackle this 'wicked' and intransigent social policy issue.

Levin (1997: 87) has characterised the approach taken to the development of drug policy at this time, which included the creation of a small committee reporting directly to the Cabinet Office and which allowed the PM to act as gatekeeper, as indicative of Thatcherite and post-Thatcherite change within the policy field.

The level of change in drug use during the 1980s had prompted calls for action and this was summed up by Chris Butler (MP, Warrington South) in June 1989 in a debate in the House of Commons:

> In the first half of the 1980s, new addicts increased at the rate of 25% a year, so that by 1988 the total number of addicts was five times that in 1978.[7]

The scale of change was sure to prompt action and might also have been accounted for by growing public concern:

> a recent opinion poll shows that the British public believe that narcotic drugs are the greatest threat facing the United Kingdom.[8]

When seeking to illustrate the harm drugs cause, politicians and others often tell a 'story'[9] and in the late 1980s and early 1990s many drew on international experiences and

---

[6] The Ministerial Sub-Committee on the Misuse of Drugs was chaired by the Lord President of the Council.

[7] Chris Butler (MP, Warrington South) from the House of Commons debate on drug strategy. Hansard, 9 June 1989.

[8] Chris Butler (MP, Warrington South) from the House of Commons debate on drug strategy. Hansard, 9 June 1989.

[9] This type of 'story-telling' response appears common and continues after this period; thus Sue Killen, a senior civil servant with responsibility for drug misuse issues, in giving evidence to a

comparisons, with the USA providing a picture of what might happen in the UK if things were not dealt with appropriately. Tony Baldry (MP, Banbury) described the *horrendous nightmare*[10] he had witnessed in New York as the result of crack addictions and Hugo Summerson (MP, Walthamstow) talked about the *rate of killings amongst drug dealers* in Washington as *quite terrifying*. Additionally, he linked the images of drug misuse in the UK to images of urban decay and fragmentation and in this Labour MPs drew different conclusions from Conservative MPs. Conservative MPs in the same debate focused on personal moral values and were more concerned with what they perceived as social dislocation. They suggested that drug misuse stemmed from a *permissive society*, which had emerged as the result of social changes begun in the 1960s and which had subsequently led to the loss of *traditional values*.[11] (John Marshall MP, Hendon South). Ann Widdecombe (MP, Maidstone) stated that:

> *Our social climate is a product of the decade of disillusion – the 1960s – and people are not expected to bear the consequences of or take responsibility for their actions ... A natural conclusion ... is that people will think there is no real danger and that they have no responsibility to consider the question of drugs.*

She and others also questioned the role of the media, whom they said enjoyed 'glamorising' drug use and the drug use of famous personalities.[12] In general, Conservative MPs were more likely to attribute substance misuse to the general population and to lifestyle choices.

> *Drug taking is not the result of affluence totally and it is not the result of poverty totally.[It] is the result of aimlessness, hopelessness, lack of direction and lack of a feeling of a place in society. Surely these are the greatest causes of drug misuse, and are likely to span the entire economic and social spectrum.*
> (Steve Norris MP, Epping Forest 1989: Hansard)

Labour MPs, however, sought to discover a link between drug use and poverty, apparently reflecting the work of Pearson (1987, 1991), which appeared to provide evidence that *a major heroin epidemic spread rapidly through a number of towns in the North of England and Scotland concentrated mainly in areas of high unemployment and social deprivation* (Pearson 1991: 167). In 1989, Barry Sheerman (Labour MP, Huddersfield) suggested that:

> *The most party political part of my speech concerns the demand for drugs and the ways to reduce that demand ... Some of the clearest information to come out of the research into drug misuse is the link between drug addiction and poverty. The heroin epidemic of the 1980s has been concentrated in the most deprived inner-city areas. That is not to say others do not touch drugs ... but where heroin reached, it was concentrated among unemployed youth in poor areas.*

Select Committee on Home Affairs in 2001 used the same approach. Minutes of Evidence, Select Committee on Home Affairs, 30 October 2001.

[10] House of Commons debate, Hansard, 9 June 1989.

[11] John Marshall (MP, Hendon South), parliamentary debate in the House of Commons. Hansard, 9 June 1989.

[12] Ann Widdecombe, House of Commons debate. Hansard, 9 June 1989.

Thus within the debates the Conservatives accented personal responsibility and Labour stressed a breakdown in social responsibility and the impact of drug use on the community (Deacon and Mann 1999; Donnison 1991); this trajectory was similar to other policy areas.

The drug strategies that were developed can be seen to reflect the personal and political stances of those developing and deciding upon them. These different sorts of explanations underpin the debates that take place and have a direct impact upon the social policies that are created. It is therefore important for those developing policy or undertaking practice in the area of substance use to reflect actively upon their own political and personal views and understand and acknowledge how those colour and shape the lens through which they view substance use and problematic use and users.

In addition, it can be seen that public concern was linked to the changing nature of drug use and both influenced political interest. The 'non-party political' response and cross-party support for drug policy, as noted previously, occurred at a time of deep social and political division in the UK and this was therefore a highly unusual feature. For this reason we will consider it briefly below.

Critical question

» *Think through – what immediately seems to you the most obvious explanation for drug use? Is it an individual characteristic or a social effect? How might these be manifested? What sort of differences might this lead to in policy? What sort of differences might this lead to in practice?*

Cross-party support, a moral engagement and stigmatisation

Cross-party support is evidenced in parliamentary debates during this period with different approaches and analyses of what drug use is, what causes drug misuse and how it can be tackled all framed within an atmosphere of cooperation and collaboration. For example, in a debate in the House of Commons on drug issues Tim Rathbone (MP, Lewes, 9 June 1989) apologised for making a party political point:

> *I fear that I must make one political comment – the one only.*

Some commentators suggest that cross-party cooperation has been a helpful feature of British drug policy but some have argued that it, in fact, stifles debate and narrows the agenda (UKDPC 2012). Labour, and subsequently New Labour, supported Conservative policies to develop a drug strategy and commended the priority they gave to drug misuse issues.[13] This was despite a difference in attribution evidenced in the House of Commons debates and discussed above. Without such cross-party support it is debatable whether

---

[13] Chris Butler (MP, Warrington South) from the House of Commons debate on drug strategy. Hansard, 9 June 1989.

the drug policies could have been pursued as vigorously as they have been. It is probable, for example, that wider social policy areas such as prevention and education delivered across all school curricula and other harm minimisation activities would have remained contentious in a way that allowed them to be politicised and thus made very difficult to implement.[14]

As we have seen, both parties took a moral tone and linked drugs issues to wider social policy analyses. This trajectory is important and will be discussed further because it continues to affect our social policy responses to drug and alcohol use; it also influences practitioner and public responses to drug and alcohol users.

EXERCISE

» Go to the House of Commons website and look at some Hansard recordings of parliamentary debates or listen to the broadcast of parliamentary debates online for any given period – now or in the past. When you do so it is probable that you will note that cross-party agreement is a rare feature of House of Commons debates.

Drugs and crime

Clearly in the late 1980s and early 1990s there was a perceived problem with drug use. This had an international dimension and accompanied concerns about urban decay, boredom and the breakdown of social controls and community. There were also attempts to link criminal activity, anti-social behaviour and drug misuse:

> One aspect of drug addiction that has not been given a great deal of prominence is the link between addiction and crime. I do not mean international crime, but the type of everyday crime that we see increasing in the crime statistics year after year.[15]

In 1989 Sheerman went on to talk about a need to concentrate *scarce staff and scarce resources* on the *really dangerous drugs*; preceding David Blunkett in his speech regarding the reclassification of cannabis in 2004 by 15 years. He also drew on proposals emanating from the Institute for the Study of Drug Dependence (ISDD),[16] which recommended a

---

[14] It is worth remembering that it was initially difficult to get schools to adopt drug and alcohol education and prevention programmes because they were concerned that if they did so they would be 'labelled' as a school with a 'drugs problem'.

[15] Barry Sheerman (MP, Huddersfield), parliamentary debate in the House of Commons. Hansard, 9 June 1989.

[16] The ISDD was a sister body to SCODA (Standing Conference on Drug Abuse). They were the two leading national 'voluntary' organisations for the study of and campaigning around drug misuse issues – they later combined to become DrugScope.

'caution plus' type scheme, whereby police officers in Southwark might caution an offender if they were referred for treatment: a forerunner of arrest referral schemes.

Criminal justice routes into treatment and arrest referral schemes are all aspects of practice and existing interventions that are now commonly taken for granted; it is important to remember, however, that much within the landscape of drug treatment and intervention is reasonably 'new' and in the 1990s was innovative.

A partnership approach

In 1985 a strategy document called *Tackling Drug Misuse* was the first attempt at a strategic approach to the social issues arising from drug misuse and it had five aims. In 1995 in *Tackling Drugs Together* these were reduced to three:

1.   enforcement;

2.   prevention;

3.   treatment.

What was also different in 1995 was the emphasis placed on working in partnership. This emphasis was not entirely new or unknown in the social policy field, nor in the drugs field, where there had been District Drug Advisory Committees (DDACs) working on substance misuse issues in local health authority areas. These had been the subject of two reports, the first by Baker and Runnicles (1991) and the second by Howard, Beadle and Maitland (1993), called *Across the Divide*, which was subsequently portrayed as seminal to TDT (1995).

In 1991, it was reported that the DDACs were not working because the *government has shown little interest* (Baker 1991: 12–13) and in 1993 a Department of Health (DoH) report suggested that these committees should be replaced by something more formalised and statutory with *partnerships established to provide a strategic focus for tackling the problem* (Howard et al. 1993). Evidence from both documents about the potential usefulness of partnership structures indicated that centralised coordination and interest was inimitable in ensuring the delivery of a national drug strategy and keeping localised partnership structures functioning. Consequently, these features were built into the TDT (1995) strategy and in 1993 a Central Drugs Coordination Unit (CDCU) was established with a remit to review the strategy on drugs and make recommendations as to how it might be improved.

There were also reports on other aspects of work in the social policy arena that promulgated a partnership approach. One issue was community safety (now known as crime and disorder), with an influential report, known as the Morgan report (1991);[17] although it did not receive backing from the Conservative government it was popular with the police and local

---

[17] Its official title was *Safer Communities: The Local Delivery of Crime Prevention Through the Partnership Approach* (Home Office 1991). It was considered that the then Conservative government did not take up the Community Safety ideas because the report focused on local authorities as the site of implementation and relationships between the government and LAs were extremely fractious.

authorities (LAs). The community safety agenda at the time was becoming linked to the drugs agenda, along with a community approach; initiatives such as the Drug Prevention Initiative (DPI – launched in 1991 and restructured in 1995), which connected issues of drug use and community, helped to strengthen those links.[18]

Tackling Drugs Together 1995–7: the strategy

The TDT White Paper sought for the first time through legislation to create a more focused and strategic approach to drug policy. It created specific mechanisms for delivery based on a partnership, multi-agency, cross-departmental philosophy and so opened a whole new era of increased attention and focus on drugs issues by a number of key players, including senior politicians and those working within the large state institutions such as the DoH and the HO.

TDT (1995) answered the criticisms of the earlier attempts at policy and intervention discussed above by demonstrating significant high-level support. Announcing the White Paper in May 1995 Tony Newton said:

> The Government today launched a tough new drive against the menace of drugs. This combines vigorous law enforcement, drug prevention in schools, action in local communities and initiatives in prisons.[19]

The strategy incorporated a broad approach and made it clear that while it sought to focus as forcefully as ever on enforcement and reducing supply, it also recognised *the need for stronger action on reducing the demand for illegal drugs* (TDT 1995: 1), which meant that issues of education and health had also to be tackled. In this way the strategy was seen to address the social issues MPs were raising in House of Commons debates and which, it seemed, the public was reflecting in the fears expressed in opinion polls about the nature and impact of substance use in the UK. TDT (1995) had three principal areas – crime, young people and public health – these essentially followed the earlier focus on enforcement, education and treatment.

A cross-departmental approach

The cross-departmental approach was underlined at the launch as Tony Newton was accompanied by the Home and Education Secretaries and Ministers from the DoH, Customs and Excise and the Foreign and Commonwealth Office. The Secretary for Health was not present and the absence indicated that the department might not give the strategy the high

---

[18] The DPI was subsequently replaced by the Drug Prevention Advisory Service in 1999 and then was subsumed into the National Treatment Agency; all forms provided a further bridge between the centre and localities and focused on policy implementation. Their work was influential because they commissioned and produced a considerable amount of research that subsequently impacted on the trajectory of policy within the UK and academic writing on substance use. In addition, many who worked for the DPI or DPAS went on to work in the NTA and other branches of regional and central government, and many of those who undertook the research have developed long-standing academic careers.

[19] Cabinet Press Office OPSS 140/95, 10 May 1995, 'Government Acts to Tackle Drug Misuse'.

priority that was required. This contributed to a sense among some commentators that the role and commitment of health agencies to drugs issues was a matter of some doubt. The ongoing tension between health and criminal justice approaches regarding the domination of the drug agenda was a traditional one within the UK (and to an extent internationally). Health-based approaches were often characterised as inclined to prioritise the individual and criminal justice-based responses as giving precedence to the community. This is simplistic, however, and also ignores the sense within health organisations that substance misuse was a 'Cinderella' area, not one for ambitious people or those seeking to make their names or careers. As an issue, drugs were perceived as too small in budget and public health terms to be significant when compared, for example, to other health issues such as heart disease or cancer.[20] Finally, the response of health-based staff to substance misusers has always included those who perceive drug dependency as a self-inflicted harm which should not be given priority in comparison to the 'truly' sick.[21] As we have seen, some areas of health and social care have historically become morally loaded and other groups who can be similarly affected by practitioner responses are those who attempt suicide, seek terminations of pregnancies or want to end their life when terminally ill.

The tension in drug policy within the UK has historically not been wholly between a health and criminal justice dominated agenda, but has also been about departments deciding what emphasis to put on their departmental priorities, and individuals who seek self-advancement and who are influenced by their own moral judgements. Thus, the issues of the penal/health divide are matters which are complex and multi-faceted and which can be seen to recur throughout the strategies, but which the partnership-based philosophy sought, in part, to address.

The idea captured in TDT (1995) was that through partnership the responsibility for tackling drug misuse would be spread across a number of organisations and in such a way that its status would be enhanced within any given individual organisation and yet would also contain (or make explicit through inter-agency debate) the moral judgements that might affect practice-based responses. However, somewhat strangely, although substance misuse policy and research gave many in policy, practice and academia a route to advancement at this time, the debates about health and/or justice seem to have remained.

Prime ministerial attention and a focus on delivery

The TDT legislation was given attention at the highest level with the PM welcoming the strategy:

> Drug misuse blights individuals' lives and damages whole communities. The strategy sets clear national priorities, objectives and timetables. It offers a basis for

---

[20] Note that public health responsibility has recently transferred to LAs under the Health and Social Care Act (2012) and the central coordinating body is Public Health England (PHE); the NTA has been subsumed into PHE and retains some regional teams, though reduced in scope.

[21] The latter is not wholly an issue related to health-based staff, although it is usually more acutely realised, for example in accident and emergency (A&E) departments. During the 1980s, harm reduction philosophies were seriously debated within the criminal justice arena, including among probation and police staff.

effective action in local communities. It is the most far-reaching action plan yet against drugs.[22]

John Major, the PM, picked out the objectives and timetables, demonstrating the importance of being able to prove action and hold others to account. He had served as Treasury Minister under Thatcher and had been seen as strong at holding others to account; the role the Treasury played in supporting the TDT (1995) legislation was important (Hellawell 2002: 304–5) and they were influential with regard to the development of the KPIs. This was a direct attempt to ensure accountability and VFM, both of which informed the focus on evidencing implementation and emphasised the cross-departmental nature of the strategy. This was coordinated at the centre by the CDCU, which sat within the Cabinet Office. In the localities this coordination was achieved by the Drug Action Teams (DATs). Reporting activity collectively was a way of tying constituent organisations into working together. Reporting itself was also a new phenomenon and one that required mechanisms for coordinating and collecting the information. The responsibilities were therefore laid out explicitly – the institution, organisation or partner was required to act collectively and individually and central government would be monitoring and auditing this activity. The information reported on via the DAT or individual organisation could, therefore, range from the number of drug misusers recorded on the Regional Drug Misuse Database (RDMB)[23] (MacGregor 2006b: 404) to a whole thematic inspection of the Probation Service by its own Inspectorate against *a number of tasks* set for the 147 services in England between 1995 and 1998 by TDT (Home Office 1997: 9).

The scale of the performance measurement, the collective responsibility and the pursuit of information by central government were new and challenging for all concerned. Clearly, the intention was that the strategy would be implemented and that this activity would be performance monitored; TDT (1995) was a clear, signposted move, therefore, towards demonstrably implementable social policy.

Partnership and local implementation: DATs

DATs were new partnership structures whose purpose was to require key statutory agencies in the localities to work together on drug misuse issues; this included health authorities (HAs) (who were charged with calling the initial meeting), police, probation, local authorities, Customs and Excise and prisons. They had 'development funds', which were small amounts of money set-up to *underpin* the local structures and which allowed for the creation of a local coordinating structure. This in effect came to mean the appointment of DAT coordinators and latterly, large and powerful commissioning DATs and/or Drug and Alcohol Action Teams (DAATS) or as in Scotland, Alcohol and Drug Action Teams (ADATs).[24]

---

[22] Cabinet Press Office OPSS 140/95, 10 May 1995, 'Government Acts to Tackle Drug Misuse'.

[23] The RDMB was later discontinued; the Drug and Alcohol Monitoring System (DAMS) came into effect in 2011 and changes to the way the information was collected came into effect in November 2012. National statistics about prevalence, etc. are now produced by the National Drug Evidence Centre at the University of Manchester and Liverpool John Moores University and are published annually: NTA website, April 2013.

[24] For the sake of consistency all of these forms are referred to throughout this book as DATs.

In some areas DATs are now combined with the community safety teams[25] but this is not always the case.

It is often hard to believe that DATs are reasonably new structures (in institutional terms) that were not initially set up as commissioners, but coordinating, strategic bodies; in general they are now powerful local bodies with the strategic oversight of drug issues and general respon- sibility for commissioning drug and alcohol services.

TDT (1995) has been portrayed as a policy success with regard to the way in which it was drafted. As illustrated, drug misuse has traditionally been an area in which there were dichot- omous views both about the nature of the problem and the best way to tackle it. However, the policy appears to have been widely welcomed and most local areas responded by call- ing initial DAT meetings and appointing Chairs; in all, 105 DATs were established across the country.

The *Drug Action Teams (DATs) were set up across England with a remit to implement the strategy* and were expected to *adapt the national strategies to their local circumstances.*[26] Given the variation in drug use, drug-related social problems and perceptions of the key issues this was a 'winning combination' and the ability to appeal to different audiences was an important feature of TDT with commentators as wide apart as Anni Ryan from Release and Alan Castree, an Assistant Chief Constable and Secretary of the Association of Chief Police Officers (ACPO) Crime Committee and Drugs Sub-Committee, both welcoming the strategy.

DATs' boundaries varied, and continue to vary considerably, with some metropolitan areas covering limited geographical spaces (for example a single London borough) while others, especially those with County Councils, cover whole counties (for example, Essex, Kent, Cambridgeshire and Norfolk). Core membership includes individuals from the police, health and local authorities (including social services and education), prison and probation ser- vices; but usually also from Customs and Excise and where they exist local representatives from central government, for example the DPI, Drug Prevention Advisory Service (DPAS) or National Treatment Agency (NTA) (and now possibly representatives from Public Health England – PHE). The core membership therefore embodies the central principle of the strat- egy – a DAT is a multi-agency partnership framework for decision-making and action.

The role of the DATs and the coordinators was to prosecute the drug strategy according to local circumstances. The strategy sought to concentrate on bringing together law enforce- ment, treatment and education/prevention agendas; how these were taken forward was for localised decision-making and agreement. DATs are therefore a policy mechanism 'in line' with the coalition government's localism agenda, although preceeding it by some 25 years. There was initial pressure on DATs to coordinate funding arrangements and some areas raised small pots of money to facilitate projects, one-off arrangements and pieces of research. Increasingly, however, central government came under pressure to develop cen- tralised funding mechanisms to allow DATs to hold and coordinate large sums of money. Additionally these arrangements contributed to a stock of debates which in turn led to the direct allocation of monies to DATs or for monies to be spent under the direction of DATs;

---

[25] The Police Reform Act 2002 allowed for them to join where desired, but this was a move strongly resisted by some localities/DATs; others did join together.
[26] The Worcestershire Drug Action Team information website, accessed 2004.

this was a feature of Tackling Drugs to Build a Better Britain (TDTBBB) in 1998 (Dale-Perrera 2001: 19–21).

The roles of the DATs, Chairs and Drug Reference Groups (DRGs) were spelled out and it was envisaged that the DATs would be composed of senior representatives of local public organisations who were responsible for the delivery of the strategy at a local level (TDT 1995: Annex D). In the achievement of this they would be assisted by the DRG who would provide the local expertise and the link to the community (TDT 1995). The strategy laid out the terms of reference for the DATs, as well as their basic composition, boundaries, responsibilities to the centre, mechanisms for communication and reporting, accountability and who they might call on for assistance. Their terms of reference included:

- assessing the scale and nature of the local drug problem;

- ensuring a 'fit' between the strategies, policies and operations of each of the constituent member organisations;

- ensuring that a DRG was established and effective; and

- undertaking appropriate action against the Statement of Purpose and national objectives of the strategy in the light of local need. (TDT 1995: 58)

The strategy allowed for prior arrangements that fitted with the new vision to be incorporated. These features have remained essentially unchanged.

The Chairs of DATs were, in the initial stages, filled by those from HAs, although Chairs also included Directors of Social Services, Chief Executives of Local Authorities and Chief Constables. They were required to report on the establishment of the DAT within five months of launch and it was explicitly stated that the agenda should not be *health-led* but that all *three strands are interdependent and of equal importance* (TDT 1995: 58). The role of the DAT Chair was influential in shaping and driving the nature of the DAT in the local area and Chairs were initially drawn from very senior ranks as a direct result of government expectation, based on the assumption that the only person who could make something happen in an organisation was the person at the very top (Mounteney 1996). As Leader of the House and responsible for TDT (1995) Tony Newton put a significant amount of energy into supporting DAT Chairs and visited local areas and held meetings with them about the implementation of the drug strategy. The CDCU also liaised closely with local areas and held conferences and events aimed at sharing good practice and disseminating information. The strategy provided an opportunity for those in localities to have close and direct contact with the centre through the prosecution of the strategy; although for some with considerably devolved powers (for example Chief Constables of Police), they were more directly accountable to the centre for their activity on drug issues than the main areas of their operation.

DRGs varied considerably across the country, in number, structure and make-up (Duke and MacGregor 1997: Mounteney 1996). They could be based on geographical boundaries, the three target areas for the strategy or composed of co-opted members where necessary. The involvement of the 'community' was often limited, with few examples which met Anni Ryan's hopes of direct involvement of user groups in DRGs.[27] In fact, the involvement of the voluntary sector and communities proved controversial; for example, some DAT members felt it

---

[27] This is an area explored in research undertaken with DATs by the author and written about in Arnull (2007).

was inappropriate for commissioners of services and those being commissioned to sit on the same body (Mounteney 1996).[28]

The DAT coordinator was most often housed in the same organisation as the Chair; those from health management, professional or managerial backgrounds, probation officers and those from local authority management structures were most common. This range of expertise had been supported by the strategy where it was outlined that it was not envisaged that this role would be filled solely by a *health service employee* (TDT 1995: 2).

In this way, as in so many other aspects of the local implementation strategy, TDT (1995) allowed for the continuation of existing and effective arrangements, but was also structured to ensure change. The range of professional groups and the high levels of seniority combined with the collective reporting meant that at the centre and in the localities traditional routes and identities were challenged or usurped and a partnership style of working reinforced.

The community and partnership

The role for communities and the part they were to play in the drug strategies is an interesting one. There was often mention of the necessity for their involvement, but a much less clear focus on how they might be included. As we have seen DRGs rarely directly included them, although they might include representatives such as councillors. The DPI focused on communities via their support for small, localised projects, although review of their functioning suggested that this engagement with communities was varied and that some DPI teams acted, in fact, on a 'strategic' basis, engaging with senior policy-makers at a local level (Williams 1998). This may have been because, as the research also reported, the DPI teams' links with the community could be a *double-edged sword* (Williams 1998: 70).

It is hard to disentangle what those pushing for 'community' involvement really meant and it was a word used by those from all sides of the political spectrum and differing 'pressure' groups. Drug misuse strategies have been portrayed, as 'apple pie and motherhood' – something that is indisputably a 'good thing', and 'community' often fulfils a similar role. This function of the term was noted in a report by Duke et al. (1995: 10) as relevant in an era of considerable political tension. However, they also noted that the notion of community, and what constituted one, was an increasingly contested sphere with a variety of meanings attributable to it and warned against the *tendency to focus on particular communities*, especially those who were poor or deviant (Duke et al. 1995: 11).

Concessions were offered to the social and environmental 'lobby' through the acknowledgement that the strategy would also be linked to *other Government policies and programmes, such as those concerned with housing, employment and economic regeneration* (TDT 1995: 54). It was asserted that these issues were not *primarily directed to drug misuse problems* but might *nevertheless help to deal with them* (TDT 1995: 54). In this too, TDT (1995) managed to demonstrate its ability to cross over difficult political boundaries and disputes, which ensured that the policy continued to be cross-party and cross-departmental, drawing on the broad range of political, social and activist opinion needed for it to be implemented effectively. Under New Labour and subsequent strategies, the view of a wider community who were also harmed by drug misuse became more powerful and pervasive.

[28] As a DAT coordinator I was personally party to these sorts of conversations and aware of the controversy at that time.

Concluding remarks

The evaluations of the TDT (1995) strategy influenced New Labour and led to TDTBBB (1998), which built on the basic structure and placed an increased emphasis on implementation. The changes they wrought were to:

*   increase the managerial and centralised aspects of the strategy;

*   increase the level of funding;

*   strengthen changes to the 'architecture' of the policy.

EXERCISE

Find out about the DAT, DAAT or ADAT in your local (work or home area) – does it deal with drugs and alcohol? Is it combined with the community safety team/remit? What is its principal remit? How does it describe drug use in its area? What size is it in terms of budget and staff composition? Who does it liaise with? In which agency is it housed? How does it talk about drug and alcohol issues? What conclusions do you draw about which professional groups influences or dominate this DAAT? Which services/agencies does it commission?

3 Social policy: drugs and alcohol post-1998

Introduction

This chapter builds on Chapter 2 and focuses on drug and then alcohol policy post-1998; thus the first strategy considered is Tackling Drugs to Build a Better Britain (1998). The strategy was New Labour's, and we consider how the party's wider social policy analysis affected and shaped drug strategy. We also look at recurring themes and consider how the basic architecture of TDT (1995) has endured. Finally we look at subsequent drug and alcohol policy, including the increasingly emergent and urgent nature of the latter. We also consider apparent changes in focus such as PbR, a loss of central direction and a move towards what is argued to be a 'recovery'-based agenda.

At the end of the chapter you will be briefly introduced to other current policy directions and debate in order to facilitate the adoption of a critical approach. As previously discussed, this means developing an understanding of how culture, history and social and political factors affect policy structures and practice. This will lead us directly into the next chapter and the consideration of the social, cultural and legal context of substance use.

LEARNING OUTCOMES

By the end of this chapter you should be able to:

» Consider critically the development of drug and alcohol policy post-TDT (1995).

» Demonstrate a critical understanding of how theoretical frameworks and analysis impact upon the development and trajectories of substance use policy.

Tackling Drugs to Build a Better Britain, 1998–2002: the strategy

TDTBBB (1998) was influenced by the changing nature of drug misuse and welfare provision, the moralised political agenda, and the growth of managerialism and partnership; in addition the emphasis of the drug strategy was subtly but perceptibly altered. This included:

- a strengthened link between drug misuse and crime;

- a greater emphasis placed on Class A drug use;

- links that suggested that both of the above points contributed towards the decay of and disruption experienced in communities;

- an enhanced emphasis on the community, which provided another strong discourse alongside that of partnership.

In addition, the partnership approach embodied in TDT (1995) was expanded and incorporated into a whole series of other initiatives that had nothing to do with drug use. These were, however, concerned with other complex social policy areas where a number of agencies were involved; so-called 'wicked' areas. This proliferation led some academics to suggest that there was an observable change in the nature of *governance* from that period and that it might be possible to trace the emergence of new institutional forms (Newman 2001). It is possible to see this change, especially at local level, although at a central level the old institutions (despite their monolithic structures being broken up – for example, the HO became the Home Office and Ministry of Justice) have reasserted themselves and seem largely untroubled by the newer partnership forms of working. Nonetheless, in historical and social policy terms these changes remain relatively new and thus it is probably too early to be sure whether or not the institutional nature of governance has been irrevocably changed (Arnull 2009; Hill and Hupe 2006; Davies 2005; Lowdnes 2005; Newman 2001).

New Labour placed *an increased emphasis on implementation* and evidencing it through the development and use of tighter performance management structures (Arnull 2009; Hill and Hupe 2006; Lowdnes 2005; HM Government 1999); those structures also gave central government an opportunity to more closely oversee implementation (Hill and Hupe 2006; Davies 2005). Again this was also mirrored in other social policy areas and built into devolved government functions such as government offices and 'ad hoc' structures such as a specially created 'special health authority', the NTA. This body has subsequently been hailed as extremely successful at coordinating and disseminating evidence-based drug policy and practice by some commentators (for example David Nutt speaking at the British Library, 18 March 2013; UKDPC 2012); despite this it will be merged in 2013 into PHE under the coalition government's cutbacks to the public sector.

Tackling drugs under New Labour: a 'new angle'

New Labour needed a *new angle* (Hellawell 2002: 295) and brought in a Drugs Czar, an increased emphasis on treatment, an enhanced role for DATs and a new emphasis on social and environmental factors. The appointment of a Drugs Czar[1] was a direct borrowing from the USA and short-lived, in part because a senior political appointment did not sit well in a UK political landscape dominated by a powerful Civil Service who essentially isolated and emasculated the Czar and his deputy (Hellawell 2002; Blunkett 2006). This was despite the fact that Keith Hellawell had been around the drugs world for some time, had sat on the ACMD and as Chief Constable of West Yorkshire acted as spokesperson for ACPO on drug issues.

The need for a Drugs Czar to drive forward the strategy was, at the time, debatable and New Labour's apparent 'discarding' of the Czar by 2002 lent credence to this view. The Czar was to have *no new resources ... no specific powers to change or challenge practice or resources* (Druglink 1997) and thus it was an unusual appointment; it combined seniority and power-lessness (Hellawell 2002).

A moral engagement: respect, communities, drugs and crime

Another part of the 'new angle' taken by New Labour with regard to the development of their strategy was their analysis of substance misuse issues. The result was a more explicit emphasis on social and environmental factors. These were approached from an ideological perspective which placed philosophies focusing on communities at its heart; an ideology that was linked to communitarianism (Etzioni 1993).

The approach undertaken by New Labour in 1998 was, in part, supported by research evidence, which at that time was emergent and the emphasis would be subsequently strengthened over the period; this linked drug use and criminal activity and made the assumption that attempts to fight crime needed also to tackle drug use. New Labour used this 'evidence', as a *validation of the ethos and direction of the government's new drugs strategy'.*[2] Of the four main findings highlighted in a press release by Tessa Jowell from the DoH about the findings from the third National Treatment Outcome Research Study (NTORS) Bulletin (1998), three highlighted gains made as the result of treatment and the fourth drew on the *savings to society* that resulted from a reduction in criminal activity following treatment – it used what came to be a powerful and often quoted figure:

> The estimates suggest that for every extra £1 spent on drug misuse treatment, more than £3 is saved on costs of crime.[3]

The impact of this direction on approaches to drug users is considered further in the following chapter.

---

[1] The title was in fact the UK Anti-Drugs Coordinator but the post was commonly referred to as the Drugs Czar, also sometimes spelt Tsar.
[2] Tessa Jowell, 27 April 1998, Department of Health News Release.
[3] Tessa Jowell, 27 April 1998, Department of Health News Release.

EXERCISE

» Complete this exercise: think of the drug users you have known/worked with and complete the table:

Name/ref	Drug/alcohol use not linked to crime – describe briefly	Drug/alcohol use linked to crime – describe briefly	Be explicit, factual and accurate – if there was a link what was it?

TDTBBB: the partnership approach continues

The new drug strategy retained the notion of 'partnership', which was described as *essential*,[4] and this included ensuring a consistency of message and action across a range of government, statutory and voluntary sector agencies, community groups and individuals. Furthermore, DATs provided a link between the centre and localities with an increasing control over budgets and widening spheres of influence; they were ... *the critical link in the chain, ensuring that the strategy is translated into concrete action* (TDTBB 1998: 3).

However, despite clearer and more direct forms of communication the tensions between the centre and localities over ownership and control of policy-making and implementation continued. Thus although *DATs were also given more control over spending*, doing so was *resisted by civil servants in Whitehall*, in part because it now made them *a powerful link in implementing the drugs strategy in the UK* (Hellawell 2002: 323). The leaders of New Labour had spent much time in opposition and understood local government and policy implementation mechanisms at a local level. They used this knowledge to their advantage in policy implementation and strengthened mechanisms in the centre that linked to localities (Arnull 2007; Blunkett 2006; Davies 2005; Glendinning et al. 2002).

The role of DATs as the implementation arm of the strategy became explicit under TDTBBB (1998). They became both the strategic coordinator of all activity aimed at combating drug use at a local level, the principal mechanism for communication between the centre and localities about this work and the means through which expenditure was channelled, monitored and outcomes reported. Their role was therefore strategic, but one also concerned with resourcing and monitoring anti-drugs activity; this activity was intended to take place in terms of the aims of the policy:

- working with communities to reduce drug-related crime and stifle availability of drugs on the streets;

- assisting young people to resist drugs;

- facilitating treatment that helped people to overcome drug problems.

[4] Ann Taylor, Statement on TDTBB to House of Commons, 27 April 1998; printed speech as distributed with news release package by Cabinet Office Press Office.

Post-TDTBBB (1998) DATs expanded significantly and became much larger bureaucratic structures, perhaps forever changing the nature of existing institutions through their embodiment of partnership and in so doing arguably becoming institutions in themselves.

TDTBBB: the language of toughness and an environmental framework

The new strategy was similar to other New Labour social policy areas in using the language of action and toughness, as well as prevention. The ideas that recur across social policy areas are those of partnership, respect and prevention and are ones which will be familiar to many readers; they are common within drug policy, but also feature strongly across the health and social care policy spectrums, as well as those of youth and adult offending (Fox and Arnull 2013; Glendinning et al. 2002).

TDTBBB (1998) heralded *piloting drug treatment and testing orders for offenders* and reducing drug misuse with an emphasis on *shifting resources away from reacting to the problem to preventing it*.[5] Thus, prevention was also linked to crime and engagement with offenders, as well as educational interventions targeting young people. These are now all common features within the drug treatment landscape but once again it is important to pause and consider that these too were introduced during this time; many have changed shape and/or name, but remain essentially the same.

Although TDTBBB (1998) continued to say, as TDT (1995) had done, that there were no *easy answers*, the *vision* it promulgated was that drug misuse was located within a wider social policy context:

> *Drug problems do not occur in isolation. They are often tied in with other social problems.*
>
> (TDTBBB 1998: 2)

The change in emphasis between TDT (1995) and TDTBBB (1998) was not confined to a sense of drug misuse as a social and environmental problem, but also concerned a heightened sense of danger. Related to this, there was a more explicit focus on the drugs that *cause the greatest damage* such as *heroin and cocaine* (TDTBBB 1998: 3). This issue later became the subject of much debate with the government and its advisers disputing the classification of the relative harms of drugs and alcohol (Nutt et al. 2010).

Overall, TDT (1995) could be read as a discussion document which presented arguments for its viewpoint and gave reasons why it was taking the approach it did. TDTBBB (1998), however, tells the reader what the problem is and what must be done; responding to drug misuse is no longer a debatable policy option, there is a clear and signposted direction.[6] Both strategies introduced features which are now common in drug and alcohol policy and practice. TDT (1995) introduced partnership and the basic architecture and structures of drug, and now alcohol policy, which has largely remained unchanged; TDTBBB (1998) brought

---

[5] News Release, 27 April 1998, CAB 107/98.

[6] For example, comparable sections on prevention, young people and drug misuse in the two strategies highlight this – see in particular TDT 1995: 16:3.5 and TDTBBB 1998: 13.

significant funding, explicit links with crime, environmental features, poverty and drug use and mechanisms that could coerce treatment.

Updated strategy and beyond: a narrower approach?

By 2002, the ten-year TDTBBB (1998) strategy was being learnt from, built on and adapted. The new strategy retained the focus on treatment, prevention and education and enforcement with 'young people' highlighted as a priority with regard to a broad prevention strategy. On page 4 the *Updated Drug Strategy* (2002) laid out what was 'new', the first of which was a *tougher focus on Class A drugs* and specifically crack use with a *national crack action plan*, more resources, expansion of prevention and treatment within the community and the criminal justice system and, overall, a focus on *communities with the greatest need*. The strategy no longer sought to take a general, broad-brush approach, but focused on the harm of drug use, particularly within its social and environmental context, with a sharply moral tone. This was further highlighted on page 5 of the strategy, which described how the *unparalleled investment to tackle the harm drugs cause communities, families and individuals will be focused in the most damaged communities*. Further, the *full range of education, prevention, enforcement, treatment and harm minimisation will be brought to bear* (*Updated Drug Strategy* 2002: 5).

The strategy focused on an abstinence model with little acknowledgement of a harm minimisation approach: *all controlled drugs are dangerous and no one should take them* (*Updated Drug Strategy* 2002: 7). It made less of how drug misuse linked to wider social policy programmes and so was less explicitly a 'joined up' approach, perhaps *in view of the close links between drugs and crime*, which it emphasised (*Updated Drug Strategy* 2002: 62). It is not clear whether this changing emphasis occurred because responsibility for drug misuse strategies moved away from the Cabinet Office to the HO in 2001, when the Home Secretary became Chair of the Cabinet Ministerial Sub-Committee on Drugs Policy. The move may be seen as the 'sign' of an institutional 'marker' being laid upon drug policy, but appears more clearly related to the fact David Blunkett was powerful in government and wanted it; further ministerial diaries and autobiographies from the time make it clear that drug policy and its moral positioning was a key focus for the PM Tony Blair. Mo Mowlam at the Cabinet Office was a weaker minister with no particular interest in drugs policy;[7] she took a less 'moralised' stance, and was frustrated by the drugs policy area, which she saw as constantly changing, with new agendas and policies and initiatives being added and involving her in lengthy battles for money with other ministries such as Health (Mowlam 2002). She did not really want drug policy as part of her remit and lost it. The move and the reasons for it therefore also serve to illustrate some key issues both about how the direction of drug policy was subtly changed, and also about how partnership, multi-sectoral, 'wicked' issues can survive in central government when managed by powerful ministers with a direct interest, but are at risk when managed by those who are not.

In 2002 the centre remained a considerable force and the PM's power and influence was a key feature. For some localities, such as the London Borough of Camden for example, their

---

[7] She had great success as Northern Ireland Minister, but was replaced by another powerful associate of Blair's, Peter Mandelson.

delivery against agendas such as drugs and community safety brought considerable central government recognition and substantial benefits. Furthermore, members of Blair's delivery unit were frequently present at DAT and community safety meetings in order to understand the complexities and garner evidence about implementation of central government policies at a local level (unattributable source: Arnull 2007).

The reasons for the change of overall responsibility for the strategy from Cabinet Office to the HO are unclear. It could have been the result of powerful personal political alliances; alternatively, it may show an increasing penalogical analysis of the drugs agenda. However, the creation of the NTA and the significant resourcing of treatment options suggested that treatment remained a key feature of drugs policy throughout this period (NTA 2013; Seddon et al. 2012). Additionally, the Police Reform Act (2003) had suggested a merging between the drugs and crime agendas at a local level, but this was effectively resisted by most DATs and the structures remained independent although 'joined up'. The picture is therefore complex and it may be that only a historical perspective will allow for clearer insight (Arnull 2013a; Farrell and Hay 2010; Levin 1997).

Thus, drug policy (and subsequently alcohol policy) moved from a strategic, coordinating central department to a large, powerful ministry, the HO; as a result it has become the subject of some debate as to whether, or not, the agenda and its focus became more closely aligned with crime and justice. The location was criticised by the UKDPC (2012: 16) in their final report, suggesting that it *encourages a view of drugs as a crime issue rather than a health matter*. This is simplistic, however, and other commentators have outlined the huge health and treatment gains made (NTA 2013); it should also be recalled that under Health 'ownership' there had not been a clear strategy, there was little epidemiological work and there was also a moralised stance towards drug users, which affected access to treatment.

There had been good reasons to adopt a cross-departmental approach in the UK and this can be seen to have worked with some success and ensured buy-in from a range of powerful ministries – a key factor in addition was a powerful lead figure who could, and would, prosecute the strategy. Under New Labour the level of funding allocated to tackle drug misuse increased considerably and resources were strongly linked to monitoring and performance. Partnership remained a key feature and at a local level DATs were strengthened through an increasing level of funding. They also became subject to much greater external scrutiny with a growing number of regional organisations with which they liaised. By 2002, DAT links to the centre were managed by the regionalised drug teams and the regionalised NTA. This undoubtedly increased bureaucracy, but the combination of local, regional and central coordination appears to have led to significant improvements in reducing drug-related harms, reducing the levels of drug trying and significantly increasing access to treatment and improvements in those treatment services (NTA 2013; UKDPC 2012).

The NTA ceased in 2013 with its responsibilities being absorbed into the newly created central body, PHE,[8] alongside the transfer of responsibilities for public health to LAs. Regional

---

[8] PHE's own website says this about the organisation: 'PHE has been established to protect and improve the nation's health and wellbeing and to reduce inequalities. It will lead on the development of a 21st-century health and wellbeing service, supporting local authorities and the NHS to deliver

structures have in general been abolished by the coalition government, although PHE has retained a reduced regional team, which it says will advise on drug and alcohol misuse. Somewhat strangely, therefore, drug misuse issues will be the responsibility of localities within a public health agenda, advised by a central, newly created public health advisory body, while belonging institutionally at a national, policy level to the HO; this is considerably more complex than the UKDPC (2012) quote would suggest and it remains to be seen how this will work and what impact it will have on drug policy in the UK.

Drugs: Our Community, Your Say, 2007 – a consultation

Prior to their launch of a further drug strategy in 2008 New Labour embarked on a big consultation, with the document entitled *Drugs: Our Community, Your Say* (July 2007). It outlined progress to date against the Updated Drug Strategy (2002) and considered areas for future focus. The title was interesting, placing 'community' right at the heart of the drugs issue and in this it demonstrated continuity with New Labour concerns since 1997. The consultation document highlights the expansion in treatment services since 1998 and says that *drug treatment is the cornerstone of the present drugs strategy* (2007: 15) and in this it challenges the notion that New Labour was only interested in drug policy from a penalogical perspective.

Public comment on the consultation document acknowledged progress (DrugScope 2007; UKDPC 2007) but called for *much greater emphasis on drug misuse as a public health issue* (DrugScope press briefing, 2007). And UKDPC (2007) in their response focused on the need for the forthcoming strategy to build on and incorporate the gathering of 'evidence' about 'what works' in tackling substance misuse.

Coalition and drugs: the Drug Strategy, 2010

The coalition government announced its Drug Strategy in 2010, which focused on encouraging people to lead healthy lives and used the increasingly fashionable language of 'recovery';[9] essentially, however, it retained the now long-standing three 'branches' of drug policy – education, health and crime. The strategy recognised that education remained important because although drug use was continuing to fall, there were new challenges, including 'legal highs'.[10]

In addition, in an early review of the strategy just a year later we were told there was to be a refocusing of the Border Agency[11] (now Home Office) against drug trafficking; alongside this a new crime agency was announced aimed at international drug supply and organised criminality called the National Crime Agency (NCA). In this too, therefore, there were features of

the greatest possible improvements in public health. It came into being in April 2013.' www.nta.nhs.uk accessed 9 April 2013.

[9] We will discuss recovery and associated approaches in Chapter 6 – 'Approaches to substance use'.

[10] Or New Psychoactive Substances (NPS).

[11] Created in 2008 from previously separate organisations and activities: HM Revenue and Customs, UK Visas and Border and Immigration Agency. On 1 April 2013 the Border Agency was abolished and absorbed back into the Home Office with two separate functions – visas, etc. and border control.

past drug policy – a fast-paced changing scene with lots of new features, names and terms – many in response to the fast changing drug scene itself.

In terms of treatment, while the language of recovery was newly used, the means of delivering treatment had become linked further to conceptions of VFM and a new means of tracking and monitoring spend and efficiency – through the introduction of PbR initiatives. The assumption is that this will lead to a focus on outcomes of treatment, not the mechanisms of delivery – thus, not how treatment is delivered or by whom. The drive again appears to be both a liberal one, ie loosening any form of central control and increasing the diversity of suppliers. However, PbR models require significant investment by the provider in the first instance before they can receive payment and thus the impact of this approach on the voluntary and charitable sector who provide many drug services is as yet unknown. The model in other areas in the early stages appears to be favouring large private sector suppliers who can afford the initial investment, for example welfare to work schemes and probation proposals. Early indications regarding welfare to work schemes undertaken by Armstrong et al. (2011) suggest an impact on the market structure and with regard to performance-related funding found that:

> The move toward outcome-related funding appears to be having a positive impact on the culture of some FND prime providers and subcontractors by increasing the focus on more targeted outcome activity. Despite this, subcontractors are generally more aware of the negative impacts of moving toward outcome-related funding than the positive, specifically noting reduced revenue and an increasing uncertainty in the market.

Despite apparent rhetoric, the coalition government has retained many features of previous policies within the PbR frameworks, but also appears to have built on these and sought to use them to even greater effect. Thus, the PbR pilots launched in April 2012 were to run for two years and to be evaluated as they progressed; this effectively requires high levels of performance measurement by the provider in order to demonstrate effect in order to receive payment. In addition they move the upfront provider costs from the state to the treatment provider thus potentially cutting state costs if the substance user does not successfully complete treatment and adhere to that for six months and if they do, the state has only paid for 'successful' treatment thereby obtaining 'value for money'. This is premised on the basis that PbR effectively links payment for treatment providers to the numbers of people who leave their treatment who are still drug free (or non-dependent) within six months of that date. Thus, there is a clear trajectory around evidencing costs and outcomes, obtaining VFM and measuring performance, all of which were seen in TDT (1995); the research by Armstrong et al. (2011) indicates that some of the effects can be observed in the welfare to work schemes and noted an increased focus on outcome-focused work.

Treatment providers are now operating at a time of increasing costs, for example heating and travel, but despite this and the introduction of these new initiatives the

> Pooled Treatment Budget (PTB) in England remained at £406.7m for 2012/2013, with the formula for the allocation of the money now including a recovery element based upon the number of people leaving treatment free from dependency and not representing within six months.
>
> (DoH Focal Point Report 2012)

The EMCDDA (2012a) has raised concerns about these budget cuts and what may result from them in terms of impacts on substance use, treatment provision and outcomes.

Interestingly, initiatives such as PbR also appear to have reverted to a more limited, individualised concept of drug use: that it is simply 'treatable'. In so doing they appear to retreat from concerns about structural and environmental factors – namely the social, economic and other forces that impact on and affect or contribute to drug use (see earlier discussions in the chapter). In this they show some continuity with earlier Conservative analyses demonstrated in the language of TDT (1995) and appear to presuppose that drug use can simply be 'treated' by a treatment agency and thus that access to housing, wider healthcare, employment, leisure, education and other opportunities will not impact 'recovery'; that is unless those purchasing services or providing PbR schemes have purchased holistic, environmentally influenced packages as Medications in Recovery appears to suggest. There are contained within current policy, therefore, directions that appear at odds with one another and which we will consider further in later chapters.

The development of PbR approaches and the debate about them is interesting and emergent in the UK substance use policy and treatment scene. PbR appears to step away from TDTBBB's (1998: 12) assertion that *drug problems do not occur in isolation*. In so doing it may also seek to minimise or deflect attention from any future potential increases in drug use from the impacts of a serious world economic downturn because responsibility lies with the effectiveness of the inputs from the treatment provider and is not linked to the deep cuts in public services undertaken by the coalition government, which are the most severe since the Second World War, amounting to approximately 19 per cent of all government department budgets (BBC 2012). The coalition's drug and alcohol strategy as premised on PbR appears to have changed the underlying analytical premise and therefore focus, despite (or perhaps because of) knowledge of the growth in drug use in the UK in the last serious economic downturn in the 1980s (Pearson 1991). The approach also belies the concerns of the UKDPC about the strategy – *there are reasons to be concerned that the approach it takes is simplistic* (2012: 76) as drug use must be addressed in relation to other *social, economic, and cultural issues* and that failing to do so potentially *restricts the ability of policymakers and practitioners to produce cost-effective and long-lasting change*. As the UKDPC have also highlighted as a 'Key Point':

> *Debates about drug policy, and policy itself, can be more productive when based on shared goals and taking account of all the consequences of policies.*
>
> (2012: 74)

The Drug Strategy (2010) has therefore demonstrated a subtle shift; it reflects the continuities in drug policy, representing both what had been successful – the three-branched focus – and a range of responses which had evolved; but it also strongly suggests what has changed, and that is an apparent turning away from a wider environmental focus which is not in keeping with its stated theoretical orientation towards a recovery model.

Furthermore, although DATs have remained in place as the arm of local implementation there are concerns that real gains may be lost. In the spirit of the coalition government's 'rolling back' of red tape and championing of localism DATs appear to be allowed more freedom to decide local arrangements in conjunction with the overall drivers of the policy – thus PbRs.

However, UKDPC (2012) and other commentators such as Nutt (British Library, 26 March 2013) have sounded notes of caution, arguing that too much local innovation may mean that real, past gains will be lost and that with a lack of monitoring and advice provided by the NTA it will be difficult for the government to evidence the success, or otherwise, of its drug policy. This perhaps presupposes that the PbR will not be used to demonstrate this – but it is highly probable that they will and this in itself has the potential to limit the scope and overall sense and efficacy of drug policy.

No government likes to recognise the successes of previous ones, but we should pause to consider that drug use has been and continues to fall in the UK; this is across all age groups – including first drug trying (EMCDDA 2012b; DoH: 2012c). It would therefore seem probable that the successive drug policies from TDT (1995) have had some effect. 'Hard' drugs with serious health and social policy consequences, like heroin and crack cocaine, have shown repeated and continuous falls with low levels of HIV infection stabilised over a number of years and a continued fall in drug deaths (by 8 per cent 2011 compared with 2010). Crime linked to drug use also fell overall in the UK, although this really represented a larger fall in England and small rises in Scotland and Northern Ireland. The reasons for this are not yet understood, but it is possible we are seeing the early effects of the economic downturn in more economically exposed parts of the UK (DoH 2012c).

Working in partnership: drug and alcohol policy – Alcohol Strategy 2012

Over the years approaches to alcohol use have become more closely aligned with concerns about drug use;[12] in part it is perhaps because both drugs and alcohol have become more likely to be treated by the same agencies and culturally increasingly used together (Measham and Brain 2005). Both also now sit within the remit of DATs and the alcohol agenda has aligned DATs ever more closely with community safety issues because of responsible drinking, licensing of pubs and other places for drinking alcohol and the management and control of the streets and public places at night.

In addition, both issues have continued to be linked to 'public' health issues and this has grown in explicitness. As we have seen for drug issues in the 1990s the public health concerns were to do with links to HIV/AIDS debates and infection and transmission rates. Now in 2013 the public health concerns focus on alcohol use, obesity, diabetes and admissions to A&E and more generalised hospital treatment for dependency-related issues (Alcohol Strategy 2012).

As before, the cross-cutting nature of these issues brings together professionals both within the community safety and public health remits who have similar and dissimilar views and raise morally loaded questions about health, individual choice and responsibility and the role of the state. It opens up the debates about prohibition and libertarianism, control and intervention.

---

[12] This is also true about tobacco to a certain extent, which is now seen as causing significant health harms and as anti-social to the extent that it is almost impossible to smoke tobacco in public places (Health Act 2006).

A coordinated Alcohol Strategy that had UK-wide features came from calls from campaigners, researchers and practitioners (for example BBC News, 10 April 2013). And launching the Alcohol Strategy (2012) the coalition government said their aims were to:

> *radically reshape the approach to alcohol and reduce the number of people drinking to excess. The outcomes we want to see are:*
>
> • *A change in behaviour so that people think it is not acceptable to drink in ways that could cause harm to themselves or others;*
>
> • *A reduction in the amount of alcohol-fuelled violent crime;*
>
> • *A reduction in the number of adults drinking above the NHS guidelines;*
>
> • *A reduction in the number of people 'binge drinking';*
>
> • *A reduction in the number of alcohol-related deaths; and*
>
> • *A sustained reduction in both the numbers of 11–15 year olds drinking alcohol and the amounts consumed.*
>
> (Alcohol Strategy 2012: 8)

As with Tony Blair before him in 1998 talking about drugs, David Cameron introduced the Alcohol Strategy drawing on images of fear and community and suggested that it was urgent action that was required to tackle not just alcohol use, but particular forms of alcohol use, such as binge drinking. This behaviour was seen as particularly related to the young, to drinking in public, to the cost of alcohol and as a new form of drinking. In this way it also became possible to atomise particular alcohol use and users and given the promiscuous use of alcohol in the UK, its deep integration into UK culture and the power of the drinks industry, this is important. Thus the coalition's policies sought not to ostensibly target the majority population and suggest that their behaviour was wrong, costly or dangerous – just that of some users. Cameron opened his foreword with:

> *Binge drinking isn't some fringe issue, it accounts for half of all alcohol consumed in this country. The crime and violence it causes drains resources in our hospitals, generates mayhem on our streets and spreads fear in our communities.*
>
> (2012: 5)

Prior to this strategy the Police Reform and Social Responsibility Act 2011 introduced by the coalition government sought to make a:

> *clear commitment to overhaul alcohol licensing to tackle the crime and disorder caused by alcohol and the resultant health and social harms, and to rebalance the Licensing Act 2003 in favour of local communities.*[13]

The focus on harms caused by alcohol had increased dramatically since the TDT in 1995 and this appears in part to have been fuelled by concerns about apparently changing patterns of alcohol use and their impact on town centres at night, the behaviour of young people and the changing patterns of women's drinking behaviour in particular (Alcohol Strategy 2012).

---

[13] www.homeoffice.gov.uk/publications/consultations accessed February 2013.

There are clear links across the drug and alcohol strategies both with the wording and imagery chosen and the methods of prosecuting those policies locally, for example DATs. However, what is different is that alcohol is not illegal, nor usually illicit within the UK. Furthermore, the drinks industry is a huge, legal and powerful global economic and industrial lobby; strategies therefore have to be found that will enable nation-states to work alongside them. For example, the expanding economies of China, India and elsewhere have led to increases in the worldwide demand for and consumption of 'luxury' products such as whisky which now accounts for about a quarter of British food and drink exports[14] and therefore has tremendous importance within the overall economy. We will consider this more in the following chapter, but an early indication of how the power of the drinks industry might make itself felt has already been demonstrated. In his foreword to the Alcohol Strategy (2012) David Cameron talked at some length about the need to increase the unit price of alcohol and demonstrated the need for this:

> if it is 40p that could mean 50,000 fewer crimes each year and 900 fewer alcohol-related deaths a year by the end of the decade.
>
> (2012: 2)

However by March 2013 in the Chancellor's Budget statement this commitment was dropped. This was despite significant opposition from some in the health lobby and the previously very public commitment to it by the PM. It was assumed by many commentators that there was a causal link between the power of the alcohol industry who largely opposed unit pricing and the dropping of the commitment by the Coalition.[15]

EXERCISE

Access the Alcohol Strategy 2012 and read at least the foreword and introduction. Reflect on the similarities and differences in the drug and alcohol policies discussed above. Think about your local DAT – does it have a remit for alcohol? If so what policies are aimed at alcohol use?

Comparative drug policy

The issues and debates about drug and alcohol policy are brought to the fore by consideration of the way things are done elsewhere and by comparison with drug use here in the UK and abroad. Those issues help to throw into relief the cultural expectations about use, policy and practice and we will discuss these in detail in the next chapter. The sorts of key issues that arise and can be interpreted in similar or different ways are:

---

[14] BBC News Scotland Business, 2 April 2013.

[15] Those who support or oppose unit pricing, however, are not easily assigned to groups (as throughout substance misuse debate) for myriad complex reasons. I therefore opposed the introduction of unit pricing and made a public submission to Drinkaware in 2013 to this effect on the grounds that unit pricing would differentially impact on the poor and the young and that we should pursue other health measures. Unit pricing and other related issues will be discussed further in later chapters.

- legalisation and decriminalisation;

- non-prosecution of drug use;

- harm minimisation and policies which support users – needle exchange, drug consumption/injecting rooms, prescription heroin, 'free' water and 'cool down' rooms;

- levels of use within the population;

- unit pricing of alcohol;

- access to public venues where drug and alcohol use is more common – ID policies, training and responsibilities of door staff;

- payment by results;

- prison drug policies.

In the following chapter we will look at how these issues affect practice in Europe in particular, where some countries, for example Portugal, have broken ranks with both formal and informal international agreements that essentially problematise drug use and retain illegality.

Conclusion: Chapters 2 and 3

The conclusion here will cut across both chapters because they are closely interrelated. TDT (1995) was an innovative policy bringing real mechanisms for enforcing and supporting partnership working across the social policy spectrum and forcing agencies for whom drug misuse issues were a peripheral matter (health, police, prisons, probation, social services, youth services, education, customs and excise) to work together. The policies under New Labour (TDTBBB 1998; Updated Strategy 2004; Drugs, Our Community, Your Say 2007) received significant additional funding and focus. Some commentators became concerned that in so doing the strategies were narrowed to the implementable and achievable, for example delivering treatment within a criminal justice setting. However, during this period drug education and prevention responses also expanded enormously with drug education becoming a standard feature in all schools.

Government undoubtedly wishes to show it achieves its objectives and this was a key factor in the way New Labour did business in government. However, one might suggest that drug policy ended up being focused on the 'same old suspects', namely the poor. Nonetheless, those responsible for policy implementation, namely DAT coordinators, supported the focus of both strategies and considered that they offered welfare alternatives, bringing into treatment the 'not so nice' drug users that treatment agencies had previously shunned.[16] Thus it suggested that the old treatment paradigms were in themselves inherently discriminatory or unfair (NTA 2013); we will discuss this further in the following chapter.

The advent of partnership successfully broke down the traditional dichotomies of drug policy because, by and large, DATs are functional and can therefore be portrayed as *new institutions* (Newman 2001) that have changed the *rules of the game* (Lowdnes 2005). There is, however, also considerable evidence of institutional resilience, with the large organisations of state (DoH and the Home Office for example) adapting to the incremental changes

---

[16] We will consider this further in Chapter 7 – 'Values'.

which partnership has demanded (Klein 1993). Certainly it is possible to see partnership forms, such as DATs, as having educated *people to see the world differently* (Donnison 1991) and thus, it can be argued, that TDT (1995) and subsequent drug policies have to date, through the use of partnership forms, delivered the innovation those designing them hoped for.

The development of the first drug policy for England, TDT (1995), can be seen to have been influenced by a number of historical social factors, such as the rise of drug misuse (Mott 2000; Stimson 1987; Parker and Newcombe 1987), concerns about HIV and anxieties about deprivation and the breakdown in communities (Pearson 1987); the last aligned to a moral agenda which focused on social welfare issues and was common to both the Conservatives and Labour (Deacon and Mann 1999; Field 1996; Donnison 1991). Additionally, international factors, such as the end of the Cold War and the apparent ability of drug issues to unite nations (MacGregor 1998), alongside the close relationship between Thatcher and Reagan, meant that Britain wished to be seen to take action on drug misuse issues. As noted above, we will reflect on the international context and the impact it does or does not have on UK policy and debate about drug and alcohol use in the following chapter.

The structure of TDT (1995) was influenced by factors such as a changing social policy agenda that sought to reduce dependence and curtail the growth of the large welfare institutions, promoting an ethos of competition and VFM (Deakin 1994; Brown and Sparks 1989; Harris 1989). It was also affected by economic difficulties and the poor relationships that subsisted between local authorities and the Conservative government in the late 1980s and early 1990s (Deakin 1994). During the 1990s and early 2000s the picture was very different: there was significant change in spend, and during this period DATs became considerably more powerful. They were also required to evidence their activity and were closely aligned to a performance management culture.

The drug strategies under New Labour had involved few changes to the policy architecture and at a local level they were essentially untouched. New Labour's analysis of drug misuse linked the issue into the wider social policy agenda and yet also promulgated a strong link between drugs and crime and linked this to community and environmental factors. The integration of drug policy into the wider social policy arena had been a new feature and yet by the end of this period it has become unremarkable. Individual agencies were held to account in core target areas, and new technology made it possible to hold detailed national data on performance in each DAT and the strategy outlined where and how it was integrated with other policy activity. Similarly, the community became strongly featured, particularly as it was seen to be impacted upon by drug misuse; in this analysis, the individual rights of the drug user might be seen to become subsumed under the community's needs to be freed from the 'scourge' of substance misuse. These are clear analytical frameworks whose development can be traced from Labour MPs in opposition in the 1980s and 1990s. New Labour's response to drug misuse was, therefore, predictable in that it built on the past; in terms of its own analysis of substance misuse, New Labour was concerned with community and personal social responsibility and their drive to modernise government and to bring about and evidence change.

The incoming coalition government in May 2010 responded to a global economic crisis by severely curtailing public expenditure; its concerns in some areas are therefore similar to those that prevailed in 1995. It is unclear what the impact of the changes will be in terms of the overall structure and architecture that has effectively supported policy. The Coalition has indicated a willingness to move away from performance monitoring and target setting; it is impossible to know how this will affect both service delivery and development. It also remains unclear whether the move away from these structures is motivated by a liberal ideology or whether it is a more cynical move to disguise cuts and the evidence of them. There are real concerns that because of the evidenced links between drug use and social and economic factors that the economic downturn will impact on the nature, scale and severity of drug use in the UK (UKDPC 2012); it remains to be seen what form this will take and how that will impact on drug and alcohol policy going forward.

We have seen, moreover, that there have been recurring policy themes, which it is worth summarising and reflecting upon. These are:

Performance management

The mechanisms of reporting and control brought positive things and could be exciting, enabling policy-makers and practitioners to evidence their work (Arnull 2009). However, they also led to cultures dominated by reporting and the coalition government upon taking up power stated that it was committed to repealing this. In part this was an ideologically driven anti-state, pro-liberal stance and in part a reaction against New Labour who significantly developed performance management systems between 1997 and 2007; however it was also in part because the culture appeared to lead to a dehumanising element (Saenz de Ugarte and Martin-Aranaga 2012). For example, it was noted in the recent Mid Staffordshire Hospital Inquiry (2013) and the Munro review of the effects of performance management on frontline child protection (Department of Education 2011) that systems appeared to lead managers and practitioners to monitor and report on activity, rather than the quality and effectiveness of that activity. It is important to remember, however, that it is not performance management that leads to this – it is the way practitioners, managers and policy-makers seek to implement it (Saenz de Ugarte and Martin-Aranaga 2012; Arnull, 2009, 2013; Feeley and Simon 1996).

Current policy initiatives are also seeking to reshape this debate through the PbR and Social Impact Bonds (SIBs) initiatives, which Fox and Albertson (2012) characterise as focused on outcomes, a lack of natural targets and a range of service providers. Thus the contention is that we are moving to an 'outcomes focused' system of delivery within the social and healthcare and criminal justice systems and away from a 'process focused' one; the ideology attached to this suggests that it will bring diversity and move risk from the state as provider to the private and voluntary sectors (Fox and Albertson 2012). These assertions are unproven at this stage and this forms the basis of much concern among current academic and policy and practice critiques of the proposals, namely that there has been little trialling of these systems (see trials in drug policy and youth justice policy) before wholesale introduction, for example in the provision of adult probation services, which current proposals would see drastically changed (*Guardian*, January 2013; BBC 2013). In all of their intended manifestations they will impact upon work with drug and alcohol users.

Harm minimisation

The sensitive nature of harm minimisation has led to a consistent pattern; each successive government has shown a pragmatic acceptance that a harm minimisation approach works, but demonstrated nervousness about promoting the philosophy as an underpinning strategy for policy. As a result, each subsequent substance-focused policy has continued to stress the importance of abstinence and the illegality and harm of much substance use.

Power and interest

The approach devised in TDT (1995), which included a direct interest by the PM in drug policy, remained stable from 1995 until more recent times with the accession of Gordon Brown and then David Cameron, both of whom have appeared less interested in drug or alcohol use than their predecessors. Important campaign groups have noted this lower level of interest from the coalition government and the PM David Cameron in their policy reports and debates (UKDPC 2012), which have received much less attention at a senior government level, while attracting significant media coverage. Additionally, there have been complaints (for example UKDPC 2012) that drug policy is now located within one department, namely the HO, and some campaign groups consider that locating drug and now also alcohol policy in just one department has had a negative impact on the policy debate (UKDPC 2012). However, as we have seen, at the point of implementation substance policy and practice are located within DATs and a public health agenda controlled by LAs and PHE.

The causes of drug use: glamour?

In 1989 Ann Widdecombe suggested that the media were responsible for glamorising drug use and thus making it seem more attractive; these sorts of images can be seen to recur in more recent times with, for example, the coverage of the drug use and then death of the singer and songwriter Amy Winehouse in 2011. The picture is a complex one because much of the coverage of Amy Winehouse's drug and alcohol use was also negative and judgemental although she appears to have died following rehabilitation attempts. Furthermore, art is a consistent arena in which substance use is explored and many songs, books, poems and plays explore the effects and impact of use. These include well-known songs that cross the generations and ethnic and cultural groups such as 'I Get a Kick Out of You' by Cole Porter, 'Cocaine' made famous by Eric Clapton, 'Ebenezer Scrooge' by The Prodigy and more recently most of the songs by The Weekend. Others, however, such as Dizzy Rascal have promoted substance non-use and have done this through comparisons with the excitement to be found in a baseline in 'Baseline Junky'.

Thus, while Widdecombe's analysis can seem simplistic – the thesis in a subtly different form is called Social Norms Theory – it is currently receiving some attention in drug education circles. The theory is premised on the notion that young people overestimate the prevalence of substance trying and use because of cultural imagery and other references that suggest that substance use is common. The educational approach is therefore to promote accurate information about substance use levels in the belief that this will positively impact trying and usage levels. We will explore this idea further in the chapter on approaches to substance use; we will also see in later chapters how there is a suggested link with cultural expectations and discussions about drug and alcohol use and their overall prevalence – this is not to say there is a link, but there appears to be an interaction.

What causes substance use: poverty?

Labour MPs, as we saw, were more inclined to structural explanations of drug use, which were especially pertinent to the forms of drug use that increased exponentially in the 1980s – such as injecting heroin use in socially deprived areas.

The blaming of lifestyle and/or poverty are recurring types of analysis in drug policy as we have seen and these explanatory forms gained increasing emphasis in strategies after 1998. They are especially pertinent in recent debates over alcohol use and in particular binge drinking (Alcohol Strategy 2012). The UKDPC (2012: 78), while appearing to take a neutral stance says that:

> the strength of the international and historical correlations between inequality and drug problems and the analysis that has pointed to inequality having a causal link with a range of other social ills, such as trust, social cohesion and mental illness, indicates that this is a relationship that should not be ignored.

They clearly do not therefore align themselves wholly with structural explanations of poverty and drug misuse but do suggest the relationship *should not be ignored* while also focusing on the psychosocial impacts of poverty.

Stigmatisation

The effect of negative images of substance use and substance users, especially those who are dependent, can lead on occasions to stigmatisation and difficulties accessing appropriate services. UKDPC (2012) have written guidance for the press aimed at minimising the harm caused by stigmatisation and in their final report addressed this issue, outlining how:

> the stigma associated with drug problems may delay people from seeking help, or cement drug using identities... It can make employers reluctant to give them [drug users] jobs, make landlords reluctant to give them tenancies and result in communities being opposed to the establishment of treatment centres.
>
> (UKDPC 2012: 95)

Relative harm

Arguments about whether drug policy should focus on particular drugs, specific users or types of use and the levels of harm that can be associated with use, have continued to be the subject of significant and heated debate. In 2009 just such an argument between government and its advisers led to the dismissal of David Nutt and resignations from other members of the government advisory body, the ACMD (Vuillamy 2011; Nutt et al. 2010). Nutt and others have argued that cannabis is relatively harmless and that other substances, including alcohol, are much more harmful; these arguments, however, can be unacceptable politically for many complex global, moral, economic, historical, political and social reasons. More recently in 2013 Teresa May, the Home Secretary, ignored the advice of the ACMD and made Khat use illegal in the UK; this move has far-reaching and profound implications which are discussed in more depth in the following chapters.

A fast changing arena

The scale of change in the use of drugs, policy and treatment responses and the scope of practice was fast paced and often frenetic during the late 1990s and 2000s and this may offer a partial reason for why many practitioners continue to feel ill-equipped to cope with substance use. It may also be why many training programmes have failed to keep up with the needs of practitioners who work on a generic level with substance users (Munro 2011). Practitioners' concerns cover a range of competencies, but have also focused on being unfamiliar with the language which surrounds drug use (for example see Galvani et al. 2011 for the views of social workers).

The level of discomfort and lack of confidence found among generic health and social care professionals may be because the language, ideas and forms of practice remain reasonably new and have not been widely reflected upon in generic social work, youth work, healthcare and social policy debates; current debates in substance use based on recovery models may go some way to bridging this practice divide as they use more familiar language across a number of practice fields, including mental health.

A focus on delivery

TDT (1995) was a clear, signposted move towards demonstrably implementable social policy and it is this aspect of the policy and the structures that ensured that New Labour used and developed them. However, it is also this focus and those structures that were criticised by those who saw the development of New Performance Management (NPM) type cultures (Feeley and Simon 1996). In turn, this appears to have been one of a number of influences on the coalition that led to their espoused 'rolling back' of red tape and centralised control. Nonetheless, these mechanisms offered ways for central government to understand and evidence what was done to implement policy and in those ways showed a stronger interest in policy implementation than is often associated with central government (Arnull 2009; Cheliotis 2006; Levin 1997).

The performance management systems and mechanisms had begun under a Conservative administration and were implemented as part of an attempt to evidence VFM and ensure that public money – 'people's taxes' – were being wisely and accountably spent – ideas strongly associated with Thatcherism. Although in a new form, which is said to be focused on 'outcomes', not 'process' (Fox and Albertson 2012), the ideas of demonstrable activity for which an organisation can be held to account continue in reality through mechanisms such as PbR. Although the philosophy behind the PbR mechanisms are strongly associated with a market-based ideology it is not yet clear how they will be monitored, nor spending accounted for.

As most social policy arenas and social policy delivery at this time remain untouched by PbR, however, the retreat from monitoring performance and reporting on the data captured is generating issues for those who are seeking to implement policy across a number of social and criminal justice arenas. Their concerns are that the coalition government's lack of focus on performance and delivery and the loss of information concomitantly leave them less well placed to put forward important arguments based on evidenced need or concerns, which the performance data would have highlighted[17] and thus less well placed to challenge cuts in public spending.

Substance use policy in the UK and beyond

Since TDTBBB (1998) the analysis of drug/crime links, social and other costs, etc. and reporting on them have become increasingly sophisticated. These are now included in standard reporting, for example the UK's report to the EMCDDA (2012a), which shows detailed and complex data sets for specific areas including expenditure; this type of information collection, collation and dissemination and the way in which it feeds into policy and practice also forms a background to current debates, such as PbR. Thus, although many features of the drug policy and its performance management and linking of philosophies with social policy directions were new at the time – for example evidencing drugs/crime links – they have become embedded into wider social policy networks and strategies and thus become unremarkable in themselves.

EXERCISE

Take a look at an EMCDDA report. These can be easily accessed via the internet. A link to them can also be found on the DoH website.

[17] Unattributable comments, Youth Justice Board Youth Justice Service Managers Annual Conference 2013; Race and Probation Conference, London, Probation Trust and IARS, 2013.

4 The social and legal context of substance misuse

How can something with no recorded fatalities be illegal
And how many deaths are there per year from alcohol
The Streets – 'The Irony Of It All'
Songwriter: Michael Geoffrey Skinner. Copyright
Universal Music

Introduction

This chapter begins with a quote from The Streets' 'The Irony of it All' because it helps to set the scene for some of the debates about drug and alcohol use in the UK in a way that is both engaging and provocative; you can access all of the lyrics on the web. As much art, poetry or song must do it foreshortens and simplifies, and the lyrics undoubtedly draw on stereotypes to achieve this too. But the lyrics also succinctly draw out the social, legal and policy context in which some substances are licit and some illicit and the impact this has. This chapter will explore these sorts of issues in more depth.

There will also be a brief discussion of the legal context and the Misuse of Drugs Act 1971 and the 1998 Crime and Disorder Act. The chapter will also look at other analyses of the 'harms' related to drug use, for example that drawn up by Professor David Nutt (2010), a version of which is featured in the UKDPC (2012) final report. What Nutt and the UKDPC propose is an argument formed on similar lines to that argued by Skinner et al. and quoted above, although Nutt (2010) and the UKDPC (2012) do so in a more legalistic, medicinal way. The reader will be pointed towards specialist texts for a more detailed discussion of the particular effects of individual substances and legal frameworks as these are complex and they are subject to change; a long-standing, reliable and accessible text is Tyler (1986).

The chapter (using policy documentation as examples) will highlight the moralisation of drug use/users and the notions of community that have formed part of that. It will reflect back on the previous chapter to do this and draw out the similarities and differences we have seen emerging during this time, and consider the move to incorporate binge drinkers and a culture that Measham and Brian (2013) have termed 'binge and brawl', a stereotype it would seem 'Terry' (as portrayed as in the song quoted above) fits. The chapter will also discuss the language around drug use and use policy/guidance documents to provide examples. This will help the reader to begin to consider how substance users are often created as the 'other' and that this can be harmful to good practice and effective engagement. It will also consider this from an AOP perspective, discussing how distancing can have a profound effect on particular types of users, for example those from BME groups, young people, the elderly and disabled.

You will also be briefly introduced to current policy directions and debate in the wider international policy world, including discussions around legalisation, decriminalisation and policy 'experiments' in Switzerland and Portugal. The intention in so doing is to enable the reader to understand the critical and analytical lens through which we can view substance use policy within a national or cultural context and understand alternative explanations and reactions.

In this chapter we will therefore cover policy and legal frameworks which seek to limit, control and shape drug and alcohol use and practice, including:

*   legalisation and decriminalisation;

*   unit pricing, licensing and other controls;

*   policies that support harm minimisation – needle exchange, drug consumption/ injecting rooms, prescription heroin, 'free' water and 'cool down' rooms, training and responsibilities of door staff at public venues;

*   payment by results;

*   prison drug policies.

LEARNING OUTCOMES

By the end of this chapter you should be able to:

»   *Critically evaluate how the social and legal context within the UK regarding drugs and alcohol shapes our conceptions of drug and alcohol use.*

»   *Critically evaluate the key debates concerning legalisation, decriminalisation and other responses to illicit drug use.*

»   *Critically analyse some of the important debates about alcohol use and its effects.*

»   *Demonstrate your critical understanding and reflection on how culturally framed conceptions, normalisations and expectations shape practice responses to drug and alcohol users and those with dependency issues in particular.*

Intoxication: a new phenomenon?

The use of various substances, be they naturally occurring or made by combining a number of ingredients, appears to have been a consistent feature of human behaviour. Phil

Withington (2013)[1] argued that seeking to profit from the search for intoxication was a feature of sixteenth-century Europe with the growth of capitalist economies and that it was from that time a global trade; beginning in the first instances with coffee and chocolate, from which governments sought to profit through taxes placed on the trade. Alongside legitimation by government of certain types of intoxication through trade and taxation, temperance movements grew – these movements usually called for the control or desistance of use of certain types of intoxicants. The reason given for these calls was the harms and behaviours which resulted, for example drinking on the streets, violence and assaults and failures to go to work.

It is important to appreciate both the historical and consistent aspects of intoxication-seeking behaviour in order to gain perspective on the nature and issues surrounding substance use and temperance movements. Seeking intoxication has been a universal, human behaviour manifested in numerous forms in most known cultures around the world. Furthermore, for many hundreds of years the movement of substances has been a global trade and governments and populations have taken a range of responses, which have included approval, licensing, taxation, toleration, disapproval, prohibition and temperance/abstention.

Withington (2013) posited that an early modern view was that it was the responsibility of the individual to achieve moderation and we have seen similar references many years later in the debates in the House of Commons in the 1980s. This has also meant that at various historical and cultural points some substances or some people who use those substances are disapproved of, as well as those who do not achieve moderation. Responses to immoderate or disapproved of substances have frequently taken a 'moral' justification and in so doing the substance user has become the 'other'; this too has numerous historical and cultural references. In the UK this moralisation has involved war and social disapproval, including the Opium Wars between Britain and China in the nineteenth century,[2] and a negative focus on the use of gin by the poor and particularly women in the eighteenth century.[3]

EXERCISE

There is a considerable body of writing about this area and this includes Phil Withington and Virginia Berridge who have both written extensively on different aspects – you can follow the references in the bibliography or search online. Additionally, if you have an interest you can follow the internet links shown in the footnotes to obtain reasonably accurate summaries of some of the key issues.

Either read an academic text on this area or follow the links provided and take an opportunity to place substance use within its broad cultural and historical perspective. When reading, reflect on and note any moral images or creation of the drug user as 'other' – think about what the links and issues are.

---

[1] Speaking at the British Library: 'Addictive personality: myth or reality', 18 March 2013. He is a Professor of Early Modern History at the University of Sheffield.
[2] www.bbc.co.uk/history/0/20428167
[3] http://en.wikipedia.org/wiki/Gin_Craze

The moralisation of drug and alcohol use in the UK: a policy response

We have seen in the previous chapter how ideas contained in the drug policies affected the ways in which drug and alcohol use and users are viewed. This included a moralised approach, which has historical resonances but in this more recent and modern context was linked to particular concerns about community and respect. The concerns in recent drug policy were, as we have seen, initially targeted at drug users and increasingly at users of Class A drugs; this approach appears to have been promulgated by particular Home Secretaries, for example, Blunkett and Straw. It was suggested that drug users posed a threat to communities and were a destructive force within them. Clearly, within some communities in recent times drug use and the selling and taking of drugs have caused real issues, for example providing alternative lifestyle choices for some young people, the growth of gang and group behaviour linked to drugs, detritus and potential harms in discarded paraphernalia (such as syringes and condoms) and people feeling unsafe because of fear of increased risk of crime and/or people hanging about on the streets. These issues for some communities were and are real, but the language contained in the policy documents, for example Blunkett (HM Government 2002) launching the Updated Strategy, appears to place the locus for blame upon the drug users rather than on the wider structural and environmental issues that underpin drug use. Furthermore, as the issues of widespread problematic alcohol use have increased, the language used about and attitudes towards 'binge' drinkers have been resonant of language and attitudes with regard to illicit drugs, and those particularly affected are the young, the poor and women.

The juxtaposition of drug and alcohol use and users alongside notions of community can be seen to have influenced and informed the debate with the resultant effect that they create conceptions of drug users (and sometimes alcohol users) as the 'other', the outsider. These conceptions are harmful and can negatively influence both policy and practice; they contribute to an atmosphere in which the moralisation affects effective engagement; and we will consider this further in Chapters 5 and 6.

Notions of community are repeated throughout the drug strategies and this began in TDT (1995), and Duke et al. (1995), when reviewing the effectiveness of DATs, highlighted that the notion of community was a contested one and cautioned against focusing on the poor or excluded. However, both in the early 1990s and subsequently, commentators have frequently enlisted the term 'community' to conjure a sense of a localised and geographically based group of people who were 'innocent' and somehow 'done to' or 'victimised'; those doing the 'victimising' were drug users and dealers and those who would disrupt the area or 'community' (Duke et al. 1995: 94). The drug users themselves were 'others' who were not generally seen as members of that community (thus not potentially the sons, daughters or parents of those being victimised), nor were they (the drug users) portrayed as a community themselves with needs which might also be locally based. In seeking to draw out good practice Duke et al. (1995: 103) highlighted the need for the community to be a *partner and participant in the process* and not regarded as *an object on which to target work*. In part this may have been heeded in the attempts to target and distance the drug users from the 'community' itself in the language used by politicians, although the impact has been to stigmatise the community of drug users and increasingly of binge drinkers.

The philosophies and approach of New Labour, influenced as they were by Etzioni (1993) and conceptions of community as something which was threatened and being lost, impacted the drugs agenda. The philosophies were in part a reaction to Thatcherism and her notorious assertion that there was no such thing as society, that it was permissible, or indeed preferable, to focus on the self, summed up in a conception of a individualised, anatomised world:

> They're casting their problem on society. And, you know, there is no such thing as society. There are individual men and women, and there are families
>
> (Woman's Own 1987)[4]

The promulgation of individualism was rife in the 1980s and summed up most baldly in the *Greed, for lack of a better word, is good* statement by the fictional protagonist Gordon Gekko in the film *Wall Street* (1987).

The philosophies of community as expounded by Etzioni and embraced by New Labour were therefore a reaction to this type of political and ideological analysis; they sought to assert a collective responsibility, a conception of society and community, but aligned these with conceptions that also placed an emphasis on personal and social responsibility. These were particularly influential and the trajectory can be observed in the following quote from Tony Blair:

> Respect is a simple notion. We know instinctively what it means. Respect for others – their opinions, values and way of life. Respect for neighbours; respect for the community that means caring about others. Respect for property which means not tolerating mindless vandalism, theft, and graffiti. And self-respect which means giving as well as taking.
>
> Respect is at the heart of a belief in society. It is what makes us a community, not merely a group of isolated individuals. It makes real a new contract between citizen and state, a contract that says that with rights and opportunities come responsibilities and obligations.[5]

This emphasis directed by the PM was consistently reinforced throughout his period in power and permeated the TDTBBB (1998) strategy. Communitarianism is said to have also influenced the coalition's 'Big Society' ideas, although their economic strategy has led to the closing of many community-based facilities which the philosophy of communitarianism sees as essential, for example libraries and parks; it will be interesting to see therefore how they will promote notions of community as their period in office progresses.

Blair also explicitly linked environmental and social factors and community issues to the matter of drugs and crime. This was a change from the TDT strategy, which had argued (as we have seen) that it was a *matter for conjecture* (TDT 1995: 54) whether social and environmental factors were more or less relevant than personal inclination as a cause of drug misuse. Linking social and environmental factors, personal social responsibility and community

[4] Interview, 23 September 1987, as quoted by Douglas Keay, *Woman's Own*. Taken from two websites: http://en.wikiquote.org/wiki/Margaret_Thatcher, accessed 7 June 2013, and The Commentator: 'No Such Thing As Society', Ghaffar Hussain, www.thecommentator.com/article/3276/no_such_thing_as_society, accessed 7 June 2013.

[5] Tony Blair, Sunday 10 November 2002, *The Observer* from Guardian Unlimited website 2004.

issues meant that the issue of drugs and crime also became a more central concern; crime to fund drug use, the impact of crime on poor communities and in addition the prevalence of drug users in the criminal justice system and the criminal justice system as a way to access drug users and divert them into treatment. As discussed, some Labour MPs (for example, Barry Sheerman) were trailing similar ideas in the House of Commons debate in 1989. In 1998, almost ten years later, they were drawn on again as features of drug use by Tony Blair in his personal statement in support of the TDTBB (1998) strategy. In his statement, Blair said that *the fight against drugs is part of a wider range of policies to renew communities and ensure decent opportunities.* This was a *fight*, which was *not just for the government* but for *everyone who cares about the future of our society.*[6]

The ideological analysis that linked crime and drug use was supported by research funded as a part of the overall development of drug policy that led to the TDT (1995) strategy. This research was known as the Effectiveness Review and formed part of the groundwork for TDT (1995); it had been commissioned in April 1994 by the Conservatives as part of the development of the strategic response to drug misuse; the intention was to look at evidence about the effectiveness of drug treatment approaches. It comprised *people from a wide range of backgrounds to reflect Ministers' wishes that the review should bring a fresh perspective to the treatment of drug misuse* and not simply reflect the views of *the drugs lobby, a self-interested professional provider interest* (MacGregor 2006: 404). The review, which was published in May 1996, concluded that 'treatment works', which MacGregor (2006b: 405) has suggested was a direct counterpoise to the popularised political phrase 'prison works'. In this sense, the review supported an approach which incorporated and funded treatment as a way of effectively combating drug use and which took a social and environmental focus. Research from NTORS (Department of Health 1996) which had formed a part of the review suggested that a substantial number of drug users were funding their drug use through offending and this appeared to provide explicit evidence of a 'direct' link.[7] This cohort study of a thousand drug users began in 1995; its findings suggested a treatment effect that was to reduce criminal activity and, by 2001, they reported that improvements noticed at one year were:

> *maintained at the 2 year and 4–5 year follow-ups. Many of the greatest reductions in criminal activity occurred among the most active offenders.*
>
> (Gossop et al. 2001: 3)

Linking crime to drug use was followed by significant input of funding into the CJS and this had a real impact upon the provision and accessibility of treatment, which we will consider further in Chapter 4.

Linking drugs and crime brought benefits in terms of increased access to treatment, but it also made it easier to conceptualise drug users as those who took from and harmed those around them – the 'community'. New Labour's structural analysis, which sought to target drug misuse as a social and environmental problem, because it was linked to moral trajectories, also led to a heightened sense of danger and of *threat to health, a threat on the streets*

---

[6] Tony Blair, 'A Personal Statement', 27 April 1998: cm3945.
[7] Whether drug use and crime are causally related or coexisting factors is the subject of considerable academic and practice based debate.

and a serious threat to communities (TDTBBB 1998: 2). The focus on respect and communities when linked to powerful concerns about drug use and structural deficits such as poverty, and environmental impacts such as the waste and paraphernalia related to drug taking, and the impact of crime, all formed a powerful nexus. The PM referred to the *fight against the evil of drugs*,[8] and talked about *the vicious cycle of drugs and crime which wrecks lives and threatens communities* (TDTBBB 1998: 1). This is palpably different from TDT (1995) where the emphasis had been on presenting a calm and non-judgemental response to *containing the drugs problem* which it too had acknowledged was a long-term issue, to which the PM (John Major) attached *a very high priority* (TDT 1995: v) and which involved government, individuals and communities.

The language, issues and context were not therefore entirely new within the drug policies, but the emphasis on threat and danger and the 'wrecking' of communities was. There was also a reduced concern with individual drug users and an increased sense of the drug user as a threat, an underminer of communities whose drug-using behaviour was linked to other anti-social and criminal behaviour (Arnull 2013a). This is a complex area, because treatment was significantly enhanced during this period and access to treatment increased greatly, attitudes shifted and waiting times dropped dramatically; however, the reasons given for funding this level of change was for the greater community good, rather than the individual good (NTA 2013; Arnull 2007, 2013a).

New Labour, in its successive drug policies did successfully bring about a change in the conception of the social responsibilities of drug users (perhaps almost more so than other groups that they also aimed at). Arnull (2007) described this as evident in her interviews with those responsible for implementing drug policy in localities and the regions. The notions that were most powerful related in particular to the impact of drug users and drug use on local communities and the findings demonstrated considerable sympathy with Blair's assertion of *rights and responsibilities* (Davies 2005). This philosophy was directly linked by interviewees to the idea of the drug user as the 'underminer' of social cohesion and support for this view was attributed by those in localities to the experiences of their communities. Those who ascribed to this view were those working within drug policy, often from drug treatment backgrounds and thus not those who one would have anticipated espousing these views. This philosophy was strongly linked to New Labour and to MPs and LAs who were responsible for poor, traditional, working-class neighbourhoods. At least some of those who were interviewed worked in LA areas, the NTA and regions where these views were common; and agreement with, or promulgation of, this view was common among those working at a regional level and coordinators who worked in large urban areas with mixed populations and income levels.

The generalised, moralised tone relating to social responsibility and drug use and used about drug users became a more ingrained feature over time and thus the *Updated Drug Strategy* (2002) contained statements such as the following:

> one single change which has affected the well-being of individuals, families and the wider community over the last thirty years is the substantial growth in the use

---

[8] 'New Drug Strategy Published', News Release, 27 April 1998, CAB 107/98.

*of drugs, and the hard drugs that kill in particular. The misery this causes cannot
be underestimated.*

(David Blunkett's foreword to HM Government 2002: 3)

The language of the *Updated Drug Strategy* (2002) is harsh about drug misuse and its social
and environmental associations. Within his first paragraph the Home Secretary suggests
that drug use affects health and family and *turns law-abiding citizens into thieves'* (David
Blunkett's foreword to HM Government 2002: 3). The link with crime is thus explicit and morally loaded; in this sense the *Updated Drug Strategy* (2002) also builds on and goes further
than TDTBBB (1998). Thus, one can see a slow trajectory from TDT (1995) to 2002 such that
the focus on Class A drugs, the social and environmental harm caused by drug use and users
and the links with crime are drawn ever more strongly.

It is not apparent from any language or arguments within the *Updated Drug Strategy* (2002)
that the changes in emphasis arose from any particular events or significant change in
drug use patterns at that time. The report acknowledges other political activity in this area
such as the *findings and recommendations of the Home Affairs Committee and the work of
the Audit Commission, the ACMD, the Health Advisory Service, the Police Foundation* (HM
Government 2002: 6), all of which shows the range of interest in drugs misuse policy and
activity and highlights how this had grown since 1995. Some of the reports were related to
the progress and impact of the strategies and others (such as that by the Police Foundation)
focused on specific aspects of drug policy such as the classification of categories of substances. The Police Foundation supported a review – in particular with regard to cannabis,
but Blunkett (as Home Secretary) suggested that *drug misuse contributes enormously to
the undermining of family and community life – more ... than any other single commodity or
social influence*. It was for this reason, he said, that *'getting it right matters so much'* (David
Blunkett's foreword to HM Government 2002: 3).

It is by no means certain that those within New Labour personally harboured negative moralised stereotypes of drug users and the biographies of Blunkett, Mowlam, Blair and Hellawell
(all key figures at this time) do not suggest that they did. It does appear that their concerns
were really about the communities by whom they were elected; and we have considered how
those concerns about decay and deterioration voiced in the House of Commons debates
led them to support the introduction of the TDT (1995) strategy. However, these concerns
became entangled with the language of morality and responsibility at some point; this was
perhaps driven initially as a response to New Right concerns, which were repeatedly voiced
during the Thatcher period but not apparently evidenced in the drug strategies at that time:
the effect in the New Labour strategies over time, however, was to lead to a focus in drug
policy on the 'same old suspects', namely the poor.

However, it is important not to underestimate the complexity of this picture as those responsible for policy implementation, namely DAT coordinators and regional drug agency representatives such as DPAS and then the NTA, supported the focus of both strategies. They
did so in part because they considered that the strategies also offered welfare alternatives,
bringing into treatment the 'not so nice' drug users that treatment agencies had in their
opinions previously shunned.[9] Thus it was suggested that the old treatment paradigms were
in themselves inherently discriminatory or unfair (NTA 2013; Arnull 2007). In addition the

---

[9] We will consider this further in Chapter 7.

changes wrought in the recent past have enabled better and more equal access to treatment for substance users. Over time the profile of those who use substances has become more similar and thus although there remain differences among ethnic groups and across gender, young people who have ever used drugs look more similar across most groups (DoH 2012c; EMCDDA 2012c).

We will discuss who uses substances in more detail in the following chapter but it is important to ensure in practice that you retain an open mind and do not rule in or out substance use and when it is present it is equally important that you are open to finding unproblematic use, as well as dependent or problematic use. Clearly social and structural factors will impact most upon the most vulnerable and be compounded by other social problems such as stigmatisation, racism, homophobia, stereotypical and discriminatory attitudes towards the elderly or learning disabled; it is important in practice to ensure that your approach is reflective and that this enables you to practise in a way that is anti-discriminatory and anti-oppressive.

Additionally, it was not just the UK that moved towards a conceptualisation of the drug user as 'other'. For example in the Netherlands the move across the 1990s to a harder line being taken towards cannabis use and 'coffee shops' appeared to create the tourist as the 'other' – the destructive outsider, whose visits to the more liberal Netherlands were causing disruptive social behaviour and bringing in 'unwanted' types (Trautmann et al. 2013). Nor, as we have discussed, was the concept of the drug user as outsider new – it is the emphasis that was new, both in the UK and elsewhere, and these conceptions were accompanied by moves to build in to the framework of social policies, social responsibilities that placed on the drug user a requirement to conform.

The impact of the approach under New Labour was therefore to introduce a generalised moral tone to the approach to drug users based on conceptions of community and social responsibility; from this basis it became possible to compel drug users to receive treatment (Drug Treatment and Testing Orders – DTTOs[10]) and the anti-social to reform (Anti-Social Behaviour Orders – ASBOs). This approach is subtly different from considering that this group requires 'management' (Feeley and Simon 1996).

The pervasive acceptance of this ideology may also have been the result of working in a partnership. Organisations and individuals gradually conceived of things collectively and thus philosophies could cut across organisational and professional boundaries; this impact of multi-agency working is one that is less often considered but it can be observed (Wong 1998). As we have discussed, it may also have been in part the result of a prolonged government discourse to which localities ascribed. If it is the former, it gives some credence to concerns voiced by UKDPC (2012) about the impact of party political agreement regarding drug policy and thus the development of a consensus; the argument being that the consensus constrains and limits critical debate.

The overall acceptance of the moralised approach, which talks about the wider responsibility of drug users to desist/reform appears to be further evidenced in the description applied to binge drinking and binge drinkers by David Cameron in the foreword to the coalition's Alcohol Strategy (2012).

---

[10] Known as Drug Rehabilitation Requirements since 2005 – for more information see DrugScope: www.drugscope.org.uk/resources/drugsearch/drugsearchpages/dttos

Social workers and other professional groups have also moved over time from a position in the 1980s and 1990s where drug and alcohol use was seen as the choice of the individual and of limited concern, to a position in the 2000s where drug users as parents or carers appeared to be demonised and drug use regularly assumed to be problematic (BBC, 7 May 2013) or poor parenting assumed to arise from a range of 'ills' attributed to parents (JRF 2007); an area particularly affected was child protection. Evidence was on occasions assembled to demonstrate that parents who used drugs or alcohol posed a risk (for example through the child's access to methadone) or that they would be 'bad' parents because of their use, which it was indicated led them to be more neglectful or withdrawn from their children. These issues are real, but we also know the benefits to families of being supported to stay together (BBC 2013; UKDPC 2012; EMCDDA 2012b).

More recently the latter view appears to have gained influence, in part in response to pressure from drug use experts and service users who have been able to demonstrate that stereotypical responses are not helpful, that each person/family should, according to social work values (BASW 2012), be treated as individuals, that social workers and other generic practitioners and professionals should receive more education and training (Galvani and Hughes 2010) and that treatment should more widely be understood as being effective in assisting parents and supporting resilience in families (NTA 2013; EMCDDA 2012b).

The current policy focus on 'recovery' is expected to support this trajectory, although social work concerns about risk in the wake of the death of Baby Peter in 2007 and other enquiries such as those regarding the sexual exploitation and abuse of young girls in and around Rochdale (BBC, 27 September 2012) heighten concern and lower risk thresholds. We will consider these issues more fully in Chapter 6.

'Normalisation' and drug use

Measham, Newcombe and Parker (1994) proposed a theory of 'normalisation' of drug use among young people and that has become an oft-quoted and researched concept. South (1999) and Shiner and Newburn (1999) countered the 'normalisation' thesis suggesting that even among the age group most likely to use drugs – young people – most do not do so. They proposed instead a theory of 'neutralisation' and argued that drug-using behaviour had been over-represented. They suggested that the changes had principally been related to the availability of drugs and changes in drug-using behaviour, which was really one-off drug-trying and cannabis use. They also proposed that there had been an increased tolerance towards certain types of using behaviour by non-users.

Since the counter-arguments, Parker et al. (2002) have further developed the concept of normalisation and proposed five components:

*   the availability and accessibility of illicit drugs;
*   rates of drug trying or use;
*   rates of recent and regular use;
*   social acceptance/accommodation of drug use;
*   cultural acceptance/accommodation of drug use.

However, rates of drug use and drug trying in the UK among all groups, including young people, have dropped: just 17 per cent of 11- to 15-year-olds said that they had ever tried drugs in 2011 (compared to 29 per cent in 2001) with similar falls in the number of those who had used drugs within the last year. There was also a big decline in those who had ever being offered drugs, falling from 42 per cent in 2001 to 29 per cent in 2011. Nonetheless, although drug use and drug trying have in fact decreased, drug use in itself has become remarkably uncontentious among many within the population and especially among the young.

Parker et al.'s (2002) thesis of normalisation as a model appears operant in a differential way from that which they appear to have expected. It is now frequently used as a framework for studying specific populations and cultural groups, for example those attending music festivals (Wilson et al. 2010). As a theory therefore it appears to offer a limited explanatory framework for some aspects of behaviour; but it is also a popular conceptual framework that has been and continues to be much explored.

One of the reasons for this is that the 'scale' of drug use and the possibility of normalisation or neutralisation of it as a behaviour is important within a social, political and cultural context and because policy-making must be seen to have legitimate aims and to be congruent with the public's common sense expectations. To support its direction a drug policy based on prohibition and prevention requires a population largely drug-free and concerned about a rise in use, but which is 'drug aware' enough to support policies that aim to tackle misuse and agree to increasing levels of resources to do so. Whether those resources are aimed at treatment or containment is likely to be part of the debate in a changing social policy dimension.

As illustrated, concerns about drug misuse increased during the 1980s and early 1990s based on evidence that it had risen and that the patterns of use and the profile of the drug user had also changed (Mott 2000; Pearson 1987; Stimson 1987). Explanations that featured substance misuse as a bohemian activity, solely the concern of the individual, declined and increasingly a link was made between substance misuse, poverty and anti-social or criminal behaviour and the safety of communities (Stimson 2000; MacGregor 1998). The agenda moved from one of libertarianism to ever increasing concern with risk; this affected professionals who responded to and worked with drug users and affected the policy frameworks in which they operated.

Himmelstein (1978) has argued that the repression of drug users has affected the poor more than the wealthy; his contention is that people with power are able to proscribe drugs and stigmatise certain types of drug use more than others. He argues that this focuses attention on the drug of choice and the method of use most favoured by the poor – in the UK for example this might mean IV heroin users in the 1980s who were seen as 'dirty' and dangerous; whereas the use of cocaine was seen as 'glamorous', less harmful and the preserve of the wealthy. It is possible to consider this as an explanation for current responses to alcohol use and notions about binge drinking and unit pricing.

MacGregor (1998: 192) asserted that the growing concern with drug use and risk led to a *fear of contagion and ... disorder* and Stimson (1987: 482) claimed that it was *linked to a demedicalisation of drug problems*. This change in perception and portrayal occurred under both Conservative and New Labour governments post-1979 and was allied with moral trajectories concerned with social responsibility and the importance of communities (Field 1996; Stimson 1987, 2000). But it was also linked to perceptions which allowed the drug user to be viewed in their social context and that this brought a *recognition of the influence of social and environmental processes in both the causation of drug misuse and in intervention strategies* (MacGregor 1998). This is interesting, for as this shift in perception was happening, social work and allied professionals within the community were moving to more risk-focused, computer-based work; thus, although this integrated, holistic perspective might have called for the use of social work theories that would have drawn more on the concepts of community-based work, systems and ecological theory (Bronfenbrenner 1994) what it would have been faced with was a more bureaucratic, risk-focused assessment and treatment process within the generic services provided via health and social services. This may offer some explanation for why generic professionals became divorced from and fearful of work with substance users and why approaches appeared on occasions judgemental, harsh and blaming.

We have discussed how for New Labour post-1997, the 'community' was set against the 'scourge' of drug dealers and users, the criminals who wrecked social spaces and parents who failed to take their duties seriously either in terms of anti-social behaviour or truancy. We may argue there could have been a role for social workers to have analysed and considered these concepts, drawing on their knowledge of the communities in which they worked and using the theories at their disposal to help them draw a picture for government about the reality of these impacts. However, by this period social workers had by and large retreated into offices, worked on computer-based systems and were less radical and community-focused than the social workers of the 1970s (Munro 2011).

The analytical framework taken forward in policy terms was therefore one premised on the thesis of Etzioni (1993), that communities (meaning the majority population) were undermined by those who did not accept their full social responsibilities and so placed an unfair burden on others, or undermined the positive things the majority were doing. It is possible to hear these same words and messages in the contention of the coalition government who have championed their welfare changes on just such a premise. Thus, it is not clear whether the New Labour trajectory of drug user as 'outsider' in opposition to the wider community will change as the NTA (2013) appears to anticipate as the more inclusive underlying message of the Drug Strategy (2010). Nor does it seem likely that the apparent shift in social work and other professional groups, which has seen a growing interest in holistic models (Munro 2011) will lead to a return to the community for social work. In fact current trends seem to suggest smaller statutory services with much face-to-face work undertaken by less qualified staff in privatised companies with perhaps some in charitable associations (see, for example, the proposals regarding the Probation Service in 2013: BBC, 9 January 2013).

Whatever our conceptualisations of drug users, the impact of the drug policies appears to have been to lower the rates of drug use and drug trying and thus it reduces the 'community' of drug users and might be expected to impact on any normalisation or 'neutralisation' of drug use. In addition, the success of the drug treatment strategy which resulted from government policy has led to *treatment services [that] are much more efficient, effective and tailored to the needs of service users than they were in 2001* (NTA 2013: 2); we shall consider this further in later chapters.

Social and legal context: drugs

The definition of drug misuse used here is that also used as the basis for much British social and drug policy; it was proposed by the ACMD (1982) as:

> Any person who experiences social, psychological, physical or legal problems related to intoxication and/or regular excessive consumption and/or dependence as a consequence of his or her use of drugs or other chemical substances.

Additionally, throughout this book 'drug' is used to mean a substance used to affect the functioning of the person taking it (Tyler 1986), but that has been prohibited for use by societal expectation or legislation – thus it is 'illicit'. As South (1999) noted, *the blurring of legal and illegal status of drugs is one among several thought-provoking features of the emergence of a late modern 'pick 'n' mix' poly-drug culture*; it has become even more difficult in the current era of legal, chemical highs/psychoactive drugs. Within the book the term 'drug(s)' is in general used to mean illegal or prohibited drug use; where this differs it is made clear.

Illicit or illegal drug use refers to drugs which on the whole are controlled or prohibited under national and international agreements. Within the UK the Misuse of Drugs Act (1971) is the format by which drug use is controlled and recommendations for sentence made. The Act categorises substances A–C and this is determined by the level of harm they are thought to cause; the classifications have entered common parlance as Class C, for example. The Act also stipulates the varying levels of control that pertain to each substance and says whether or not it can be used for medical or research purposes and the type of licensing required for these activities – these are the Schedules. Thus, as the UKDPC (2012) makes clear, the term 'illegal drugs' can be misleading; heroin is illegal in certain forms, when it is produced, distributed and possessed by some people in specified contexts; whereas in the form of morphine, produced by a licensed supplier, distributed by a qualified medical practitioner in specified circumstances and possessed by the user as specified by the medical practitioner it is perfectly legal.

The International Convention for Narcotics Control established in 1928 laid out the broad framework of drugs that were proscribed, although its principal focus had in fact been to control the opium trade. In 1961 the Single Convention on Narcotic Drugs was set up and listed more than a hundred substances, under four Schedules, with the aim to control the cultivation, production, manufacture, export, import and distribution, possession and use and trade of substances, focusing on plant-based narcotics on an internationally agreed basis. In 1971 the Convention on Psychotropic Substances sought to provide a similar level of control using four Schedules for psychotropic drugs such as amphetamines and in 1988 the Convention against Illicit Traffic in Narcotic Drugs and Psychotropic Substances brought the two previous agreements together and introduced new provisions in response to the changing nature of drug use, possession and trade; the changes included controls on money laundering. Within Europe there is another raft of controls and legislations such as penalties regarding trafficking and the most recent, 2005 European Council Decision on new psychoactive substances, which agreed to share information on the new 'legal' highs.[11]

---

[11] The UKDPC (2012) report also provides a comprehensive, intelligible summary of the international and European agreements and policy structures.

International agreements continue to hold powerful sway as we shall see with recent attempts to change drug laws within independent countries and discussed below. Both those agreements and the Misuse of Drugs Act (1971) are too legalistic, detailed and changing to be usefully discussed in detail here; specialist texts and guidance from the government website are easily accessed on the internet and provide access to ACMD papers, House of Commons Select Committees and debates regarding drug classifications and the details of those classifications, schedules, etc.

As we have seen, interest in drug issues was altered when the nature and scale of drug use/misuse at a local, national (Stimson 1987) and international level changed during the late 1970s and 1980s, and this presented nation-states with issues with which they needed to deal (Mowlam 2002: 367). There had been an economic downturn in the 1970s, the collapse of the welfare state (Deakin 1994; Harris 1989), a rise in New Right explanations for social behaviour, which were increasingly popularised and accepted (Brown and Sparks 1989) and a growth in crime; all were linked in some way to changing explanations of drug misuse (MacGregor 1998, 1999). There is also evidence that in the UK (and the USA) the social and economic policies pursued widened the gap between rich and poor and that this gap grew substantially between 1979 and 1989 (Townsend 1993). The impact of social policies like this was to create increased levels of perceived social dislocation and related problems, such as a growing crime rate (Downes 1995). Additionally, England and Scotland experienced a heroin epidemic that *settled with particular severity in areas of high unemployment, social deprivation and housing decay* (Pearson 1987: 94).

A link was made between economic deprivation and drug misuse; heroin, in particular, in the UK. In the USA, writers such as Eloise Dunlap (1995: 115) researched in-depth, ethnographic studies, which provided detailed evidence of the way in which: *macro level 'social forces' create conditions which lead to stressful situations and conflicts at a household level.* The suggestion was that the failure to address these fault lines, resulted in further *crisis induced responses*, of which drug misuse *is only one response* (Dunlap 1995: 117). The focus taken by some academics on specific geographical areas and groups introduced and popularised the conceptual link between community, environmental factors and drug use (MacGregor 1998).

The account of a change in drug-using behaviour in the UK (Parker et al. 1987; Pearson 1987; Mott 2000) is now largely accepted and has subsequently been built into British drug policy, along with an explanation that (more controversially) links drug misuse with crime (NTA 2013; UKDPC 2012; Task Force 1996: 1[12]). Additionally, empirical studies were commissioned and appeared to provide the evidence for this (Task Force 1996). They suggested that those who had committed offences were also misusing drugs and that there was a link between the two behaviours; driving down one would, therefore, arguably lead to a drop in the other (Task Force 1996). Feely and Simon (1996) have commented that the power and persuasion of such accounts allowed managerialist-based assumptions about drugs and crime to be instituted into the penal fabric and that these assumptions led to the identification of groups of people who could then be 'contained' or 'treated'. It is possible to see the response to this actuarial challenge within drug and crime policies particularly under New

---

[12] This was the Task Force to Review Services for Drug Misusers 1996.

Labour, but as we have noted the picture is much more complex than Feeley and Simon (1996) suggested.

Furthermore, we can see a range of policies developed that aim to tackle a whole raft of social policy areas MacGregor (1999) has argued were identified as relevant to future potential criminality or drug use. We can see some of these policies in New Labour's Sure Start for example, which sought to tackle areas of deprivation, anomie and aimlessness and bolster prevention efforts.

Because of the complexity of the targets that Sure Start type programmes aimed to hit, and because many of those they targeted were and still are young, and most were set up with local influence and in response to local needs, it was initially difficult to establish a definitive picture regarding their success (Little 2007); however Eisenstadt (2011) has argued that in combination the results show convincingly that government can no longer ignore the importance of targeted, early intervention programmes for assisting children and families affected by structural disadvantages like poverty. Furthermore, a randomised control trial (RCT) by Hutchings et al. (2007) showed the effectiveness of an evidence based parenting intervention delivered with fidelity by regular Sure Start staff, with the results indicating that where staff were clear about what they were doing, why and what they expected the outcome to be, the results were very positive for children and families – the authors argue that this entails a message for all practice.

With regard to drug use we have seen significant falls in drug trying among the young and overall regular drug use remains low, with 7 per cent of all adults saying they had used cannabis in the year 2011/12. And yet despite this the UK continues to report reasonably high levels of drug trying and use in comparison with others in Europe, with cannabis remaining the illicit drug most likely to be tried, with 31 per cent of adults in England and Wales saying in 2011/12 that they had used it at some time in their lives (DoH 2012d; EMCDDA 2012a, 2012c).

In his final report Paul Hayes (NTA 2013), the Chair at the time of the NTA, reflected on what he considered had been achieved since their inception in 2001 in the drug treatment of those whose use was problematic. He suggested that there had been significant gains with many drug users brought into treatment with proven benefits in terms of health outcomes for the drug user and social benefits for the user's family and community. We will consider this further in Chapter 5, but it is worth considering in some detail at this point what he said; it succinctly sums up what has been gained and the reader is asked to keep in mind when reading it that the UK has reasonably high levels of drug trying and use compared to other European countries:

> *The rate of HIV infection amongst injecting drug users in England is 1.3% compared to 3% in Germany, 12% in Italy and 16% in the US. Drug-related deaths have begun to fall following rapid rises during the previous 20 years, despite today's drug using population being older and more vulnerable. The Home Office estimates that the rapid access to treatment offered by the Drug Intervention Programme allied to overall expansion of treatment availability is preventing 4.9m crimes a year. Both drug use and demand for treatment are falling – most rapidly among younger people.*
>
> *The overall number of heroin and crack users is now below 300,000 for the first time since estimates began, from a peak of 332,000 in 2005–06. The number*

of heroin users coming into treatment for the first time has fallen from 48,000 in 2005–06 to 9,000 in 2011–12.

(NTA 2013)

It is not possible at this point in history to be sure which linkages, mechanisms and policies were responsible for delivering the health and criminal justice outcomes, but it would appear that drug and other social policies certainly contributed to the gains made as well as DAT teams and other actors within this policy and practice sphere. Thus Hayes (NTA 2013) makes claims for the success of policies that were delivered by partnership mechanisms, but highlights that:

By 2005 ... [it was] apparent ... the NTA would achieve its initial objectives to double the number of people in treatment, reduce waiting times and ensure rapid access to treatment for offenders ... (the) focus began to shift towards treatment completion, seeking a balanced system in which the accessibility and stability of low threshold maintenance prescribing was allied to the ambition to achieve safe, sustainable treatment exit and eventual recovery.

[By] ... the 2008 Drug Strategy ... we were seeing year-on-year increases in successful and sustained treatment completions.

He finishes commenting that *the coalition government's new 2010 Drug Strategy which explicitly committed to build onto the achievements of its predecessor* offers *a new emphasis on the individual's right to expect treatment to promote their journey towards recovery*, and which he anticipates will balance *community benefit with individual aspiration, supported by continued investment and clinical guidance.*

It is debatable whether these things can and will be achieved in a climate of significant welfare cuts, PbR and the absorption of the NTA in PHE, which has much larger, overall public health issues to consider; only time will allow us to consider the impacts.

EXERCISE

Undertake some further reading about the control of substances as outlined above and the harms said to be associated with them and then complete this table for as many substances as you feel able – cover at least five. Do this in such a way that you can add to it as you progress throughout the book:

Name of substance	Relevant national legislation	Classification under Misuse of Drugs Act	Schedule under Misuse of Drugs Act	Relevant international legislation	Harms associated with this drug	Effects attractive to user
For example, heroin						

Social and legal context: alcohol

Alcohol is not an illicit drug in that it is in general socially acceptable in the UK; it is widely available and widely used. However, alcohol is produced, distributed and sold under licence and thus it is not different from other substances in that respect. The legislation that controls it, however, is different and includes the Licensing Act 2003 which controls the sale and supply of alcohol.[13] People wishing to obtain a licence can apply to their local council for a personal, premises or club premises licence and may also need to consult with the 'responsible authorities' who are the:

- police;
- local fire and rescue;
- primary care trust (PCT) or local health board (LHB);
- the relevant licensing authority;
- local enforcement agency for the Health and Safety at Work etc. Act 1974;
- environmental health authority;
- planning authority;
- body responsible for the protection of children from harm;
- local trading standards;
- any other licensing authority in whose area part of the premises is situated.

The apparently changing patterns of alcohol use in the UK have led to increasing concerns about how, when and by whom it is used and have led to a review of the controlling legislation by the coalition government focusing on:

- rebalancing the Licensing Act 2003 in favour of local communities;
- crime and disorder caused by alcohol;
- health and social harms.

As you can see, the concerns and the language bear remarkable similarity to that featured in earlier drug legislation. Furthermore, some changes have been made already in other pieces of legislation such as the Police Reform and Social Responsibility Act 2011, which included:

- doubling the fine for persistent underage sales to £20,000;
- introducing a late-night levy to help cover the cost of policing the late-night economy;
- increasing the flexibility of early morning alcohol restriction orders;
- reducing the evidential requirement placed upon licensing authorities when making their decisions;
- removing the vicinity test for licensing representations to allow more people to comment on alcohol licences;

---

[13] www.gov.uk/alcohol-licensing, accessed 11 June 2013.

- reforming the system of temporary event notices;
- suspension of premises' licences if annual fees are not paid.

Furthermore, it would be foolish to give the impression that the consumption of drugs and alcohol have not been commonly linked. In the reality of the lives of many drug and alcohol users the two have always coexisted and there was often a false dichotomy among some practitioners, policy-makers and in some academic writing. Cocaine and alcohol, or cannabis and alcohol, are among the most commonly used-together especially since the 1980s, while some cultural groups, such as the dance drug culture in the 1990s and some 'hippy' groups and cannabis-using cultures appeared to eschew alcohol.

Measham and Brain (2005) have argued that there is evidence that within Britain there now exists a cultural norm that is about the seeking of an intoxicated state and this may include alcohol and/or other substances and that a wide range of young people engage in this type of activity and/or see it as acceptable. They suggest that this has been the result of a number of social, policy and legislative changes, including for example long opening hours. They argue that the changes across economic and social spheres can be seen to demonstrate how ambiguous Britain's approach to alcohol is.

Perhaps, however, we can consider that the current situation within the UK with regard to the complex mix of the use of appropriate legal, licit and illicit substances among otherwise law-abiding citizens also highlights some of the overall ambiguities towards states of intoxication more generally. Thus:

- there is a tension between legal, licit and illicit substances – for example arguments regarding classification and the position of 'legal highs';
- there are approved sites and routes of use and those which are disapproved – for example drinking wine with dinner – would usually not be problematised; drinking wine alone, at home on a weekday at 10am would be;
- there is ambiguity concerning those who are allowed to make choices about their state (or not) of intoxication – for example those over a given age (currently 18 years in the UK), in the past gender (ie it was more acceptable for men than women to drink alcohol or smoke tobacco), those who are deemed medically, physically or mentally competent to make the decision to be/not to be intoxicated, etc.

Nonetheless, although drugs and alcohol are frequently used together across a whole range of social and cultural contexts and across all strata of socio-economic groups, many more people in the UK drink alcohol than use drugs. Furthermore, as we have seen, drug use has fallen since 2001 and this has been marked among young people; at the same time we have seen an increase in alcohol use (see Figure 4.1).[14]

Alcohol-related deaths are said to have more than doubled since the 1990s and now stand at approximately 9,000 per year; it is wise to be cautious with these figures as alcohol-related harms were notoriously underestimated in the past as the figures simply were not collated, eg admissions to A&E which were alcohol-related, etc. Thus New Labour's focus on collating data and reporting and monitoring it made information available but could also

[14] www.bbc.co.uk/news/health-21621144, accessed 10 April 2013.

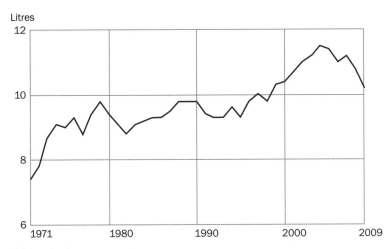

Figure 4.1 UK alcohol consumption per capita 1971–2009
Note: Figures for adults aged over 15
Source: British Beer and Pub Association

provide unwelcome news, or suggest apparent shifts in behaviour. Nonetheless, there are concerns about the level of alcohol use within the UK and the changing patterns of consumption, and as a result a number of organisations came together to campaign for a number of wide-ranging changes that include:

• limiting sales through the use of particular and specified checkouts;

• limits on the hours during which alcohol could be sold;

• similarly to tobacco limiting or stopping advertising and promotion, as well as labelling warning of the health effects;

• standardising licensing hours again;

• reducing the limit at which one can drink alcohol and legally drive.

On the premise that the lower cost of alcohol has fuelled the rise in consumption, a key suggestion was that there should be a base unit price for alcohol which would in effect be a considerable increase. This idea was popularly supported and has been adopted in Scotland, which will in effect be something of a natural experiment (akin to that for harm reduction measures which were not adopted in Edinburgh) by providing comparable data in the coming years between different parts of the UK where unit pricing has or has not been adopted.[15] Research by Stirling University had suggested that a *50p minimum price would reduce consumption by 6.7% which after 10 years would mean there were 3,000 fewer alcohol deaths and 100,000 fewer hospital admissions.*[16]

---

[15] However, it has been suggested anecdotally that while the policy has been adopted formally no steps have been or are being taken to implement the policy and thus that it is unlikely that it will be implemented.

[16] www.bbc.co.uk/news/health-21621144, accessed 10 April 2013.

The debate around unit pricing has been vociferous with strong support from some members of the medical community, while it has been strongly and almost uniformly opposed by the drinks industry who have argued for 'targeted solutions' that focus on problematic groups, individuals or areas. However, those who oppose it have been a mixed group, which has also included those who are experts in the field but who take a holistic, structural view and who consider that adopting unit pricing unfairly and illegitimately impacts the poor and the young and that there are other social, cultural and educational approaches that could usefully be taken.[17] As we saw, David Cameron appeared to give unconditional support to unit pricing and was due to introduce it, but in 2013 it was unexpectedly dropped from the budget – many saw the hand of the powerful drinks industry in that move (Channel 4 News, 17 July 2013; BBC, 1 March 2013).

Legalisation and decriminalisation

Some of the key issues that have been continually present within the substance use debates include those of legal, licit, prescribed and illicit use, as we have seen, and the changing pattern for some substances or acceptability determined by cultural mores. What this means is that people have discussed and argued about why certain substances that produce states of intoxication are legal, permitted or frowned upon or are illegal in certain cultures, countries or historical periods – for example:

• alcohol during prohibition in the USA in the 1920s;

• alcohol in some Muslim states currently – for example Saudi Arabia;

• heroin is illegal currently in the UK, although morphine is acceptable for medical use and methadone by prescription;

• cannabis is illegal but often tolerated in many states across Europe – for example the UK and Holland;

• Khat use was tolerated in the UK until 2013, but has been illegal in Sweden for some time;

• drug use has been decriminalised in some countries – for example in Portugal currently.

The differences between legal use and decriminalisation are subtle and are in part related to international agreements and international trade in drugs, which countries cannot determine solely for themselves without other consequences or cannot control alone.

It has been argued that since President Nixon began the war on drugs in 1971 the USA has remained a powerful defender of this position and an opponent of those who have sought to debate or change it. However, in 2013 a powerful alliance of American countries as part of the Organization of American States (OAS) General Assembly Meeting sought to bring about some change because of what they perceived to be the high toll in terms of *the carnage of brutal drug trafficking organizations to the egregious abuses by security forces fighting them.*[18] The impact of drug use on countries in South America has been

---

[17] I, for example, fall into this category and made a submission to Drinkaware in 2013 which is publicly available to this effect.

[18] Quote attributed to Jose Miguel Vivanco, Director of OAS; article by Diaz 2013 in the *Huffington Post*: www.huffingtonpost.com/2013/06/04/new-drug-war-strategy-_n_3383786.html and http://latino.foxnews.com/latino/news/2013/06/04/oas-meeting-focuses-on-new-drug-strategies

particularly destructive, prompting the research that led to the report.[19] The changes they sought were to develop drug policy that took a more educative, preventative approach and included decriminalising cannabis production, supply and use; they did not at this stage propose decriminalising cocaine, which causes them the most structural, social and criminal justice problems. The change in policy was not carried at the meeting because of opposition from the USA, but many felt there had been some change just in getting the discussion going.[20] Furthermore, it mirrors some debates in Europe where other countries such as Portugal, the Czech Republic and Switzerland have moved towards greater toleration or active attempts at decriminalisation related in particular to the possession of small amounts of drugs.

The illegal drug trade is controlled by powerful, criminal interests and gangs/organisations; it would not be easy for a government to be seen to negotiate or do business with them. By acting in concert such as the South American countries, they afford themselves some protection. Nonetheless many countries have been ravaged by drug production and its control by powerful criminal gangs; there is interesting work on this with regard to Afghanistan for example. In all of the instances the extreme nature of some drug production and supply routes has led to serious structural, cultural and social problems.

In Europe and the UK the extremes that South America and Afghanistan have experienced have not impacted in the same way but the complexities of policing substance use when that has become increasingly complex, or when it appears to become widespread or 'normalised' in large parts of the population are issues that have arisen. For this web of reasons and others, decriminalisation has often been seen as an 'easier' option for a government looking for a way to extricate itself from the problems. Currently, legal highs and the use of psychoactive, synthesised drugs are presenting additional and ever more complex challenges to governments who appear unable to 'outlaw' chemical variants at a speed fast enough to keep up with the drugs industry able to produce them. In 2013 Professor Les Iversen, the current Chair of the ACMD warned that the government could not keep up with the 200 or more legal highs currently available in the UK and that these posed a danger to health.[21] The Home Office has therefore introduced *temporary banning orders that outlaw the supply and sale but not possession of the drugs, pending an examination of their harmful effects* (*Guardian*, 16 May 2013). For reasons not entirely clear, Iversen has rejected the approach being taken in New Zealand to test and license *the sale of these new psychoactive substances* and appears to be considering solutions such as *tweaking the Medicines Act or using consumer protection laws* (*Guardian*, 16 May 2013).

Decriminalisation has been strongly called for with regard to cannabis use both within the UK (Transform, 22 July 2013) and globally as we have seen in 2013 at the OAS conference. The widespread use of cannabis among a largely otherwise law-abiding population (for example 'Tim' in The Streets' song at the start of this chapter) has called into question the viability of upholding a law so many disregard or have disregarded (one-third of all adults in the UK at

---

[19] www.countthecosts.org/sites/default/files/CICAD-Marketing-Document-ENG.pdf

[20] www.utsandiego.com/news/2013/Jun/07/no-drug-policy-change-as-oas-wraps-up-in-guatemala

[21] www.guardian.co.uk/uk/2013/may/16/legal-highs-risk-overdose-drugs-tsar

some time); this argument is derived from the basic legal principle that in a democratic state laws should only be upheld with the consent of the population.[22]

There is little evidence of widespread harm associated with cannabis use (for example see Nutt 2010; discussed further in later chapters) and it appeared that cannabis was on the way to being decriminalised in the UK when it was downgraded on the drugs index in 2004 from B to C following an ACMD recommendation in 2002.[23] However, in 2008 Jacqui Smith reclassified it back to B despite ACMD advice; acting in direct contradiction to scientific advisers' advice was considered unprecedented. This move appears to have been the result of the 'moral' standpoint supported by some in government, the police, the Magistrates' Association and some mental health charities, such as SANE, but was rejected by drug experts and many in the medical community. Smith said that her concerns were about stronger and more potent forms of cannabis, known as Skunk, which were increasingly appearing on the drugs scene; although she acknowledged that the research evidence of harm was mixed, she used this somewhat surprisingly to reclassify on the basis that it was better to 'err on the side of caution'.[24] The UKDPC (2012) reported, however, that during the period of reclassification down and then up, there was in fact an overall decline in use and the legal status appeared to have little impact. Currently there are claims that farms for growing cannabis in the UK are linked to organised criminality and the trafficking of women and children in particular who are forced to work on the farms (*Sunday Times*, 25 August 2013). The links with organised crime, for example in the cultivation of cannabis, for some show the undoubtedly problematic nature of substances and why they should remain illegal; for others they 'demonstrate' the difficulties and problems illegal status brings and strengthen their calls for decriminalisation.

A more recent example of a Home Office minister ignoring the advice of a specialist committee came in 2013 when Teresa May decided to criminalise possession of Khat in contravention of the advice of the ACMD; her reasoning appeared similarly illogical to that of Smith in 2008 (*Guardian*, 3 July 2013). This decision was apparently based on concerns about the UK becoming a 'trafficking' point for Khat within Europe because of its legal status. However, the decision to make it illegal has potentially serious social, cultural and political repercussions, which are certainly not commensurate with any physiological effects of the drug. Khat use is ingrained into Somali culture in a way very similar to alcohol within the UK (Patel et al. 2005). The change in legal status therefore has the potential to criminalise otherwise law-abiding people for a behaviour which they consider 'normal'. In addition, there are concerns about the potential for widening stop and search powers, which already unfairly target those from BME communities. Further, it may increase the links between trade in Khat and other illicit drug supply/suppliers and thereby expose Khat users to other substances (compare for example the current separation of cannabis from other drug markets in Holland which appears to be the result of toleration of cannabis use). While Khat use had not been

---

[22] Arguments about how the rule of law is applied and the rights that appertain to citizens and rulers date back to the Greeks and Aristotle and beyond; they continue to be of political significance, for example forming part of a debate and resolution at United Nations General Assembly 67th General Assembly Plenary (24 September 2012). Such debates are key with regard to the rights of substance users and how laws are formed and upheld.

[23] ACMD (2002).

[24] http://news.bbc.co.uk/1/hi/7845023.stm, accessed 11 June 2013.

considered to be entirely unproblematic within the Somali community (Patel et al. 2005: like alcohol use in the UK) the decision by May now offers real possibilities for social dislocation, discrimination and harm. It is very difficult to understand the decision in a light other than one premised on notions of a 'war on drugs'.

The arguments of commentators about reclassifying substances in line with their overall harms – social, economic and legal – such as those proposed by Nutt (2010) and the UKDPC also appear to have been ignored by both the New Labour government and the current coalition government. Nutt was sacked by New Labour and the coalition government has similarly ignored expert advice. The assessment is based on a range of 'harms' to the substance user and others, including social, psychological and environmental harms. Using these criteria it was proposed that substances would be classified as follows, with the most serious first:

1. Alcohol

2. Heroin

3. Crack cocaine

4. Metamphetamine

5. Cocaine

6. Tobacco

7. Amphetamine

8. Cannabis

9. GHB

10. Benzodiazepines

11. Ketamine

12. Methadone

13. Mephedrone

14. Butane

15. Khat

16. Anabolic steroids

17. Ecstasy

18. LSD

19. Buprenorphine

20. Mushrooms

Clearly achieving such a reclassification would involve substantial legal and social change and have significant impacts on the environment and economic situation. The arguments were seriously made, however, and based on evidence and assessments of that evidence. Nutt (2010) acknowledged that such an assessment has limitations, for example it is informed by judgement; he asserts, however, that the framework used to draw up the list above (and other similar lists) was constructed to minimise judgement error (2010: 1559, 1564). An important acknowledgement is that only harms are counted, not benefits including pleasure, which in terms of 'why' people choose to use substances despite risk of harm is an important factor. However, other current legal proscriptions do not seek to weigh benefit or pleasure either so in this respect the relative scales of risk and harm do not differ.

The complexities of fighting a war against drugs, for a range of social, structural and cultural reasons are such that elsewhere in the world the pressures to maintain the consensus to take a harsh anti-drugs approach in place since the 1970s appears to be breaking down. Portugal has taken the step of decriminalising drug use and this too provides something of a 'natural experiment' for the rest of the world and the West in particular. We will consider this in more detail below.

EXERCISE

Look at the classification of drugs in the Misuse of Drugs Act and look at an alternative classification such as Nutt (2010), Van Amerstadm et al. (2010), UKDPC (2012). Using the table you began to construct in Chapter 3 regarding drug and alcohol use and crime and using the same anonymised people as examples add other sections related to relative harms and benefits; complete this by being very specific about what the harm or benefit was and be specific for each substance as these harms and benefits may differ:

Harm to self of substance use	Harm to others of substance use	Benefits to self of substance use	Benefits to others of substance use

Social and legal context of drug use beyond the UK

The Portuguese 'experiment' has had a well-documented trajectory because of European monitoring through the EMCDDA and thus it provides a very real example of what the consequences of liberalised drug use policies might be.

Europe also provides concrete examples of different patterns of alcohol use and behaviour across the whole population and young people in particular and thus facilitates an understanding of the impact of culture, social and economic factors and their mediating effects. Differential effects can be found within countries, cultures, ethnic groups or drug use groups or across countries; we will look at this in more detail in following chapters, but, for example, research might focus on how different drug users might be facilitated to access treatment services by moderating or changing the services offered (Arnull et al. 2007).

Within the USA, academics and commentators have argued that there has been a continued pursuit of a hard line, 'war on drugs' approach despite high concentrated levels of drug use and significant problems focused in particular communities. The policies pursued have had well-documented differential demographic impacts: there is a large body of work on this in the USA and Eloise Dunlap's (1995) study provides a moving illustration of the effects of macro-level social forces and the way they impact on individual households; for those interested in ecological, systemic or structural approaches to practice this is an accessible ethnographic study. Philippe Bourgois is another US academic and writer who has written extensively and undertaken ethnographic studies focusing in particular on the impact of ethnicity (see for example Bourgois and Schonberg 2007); his work is also accessible and readable. Some, such as the documentary film-maker Eugene Jareki (*The House I Live In*, 2012), posit that the USA's approach, which is to fight a 'war on drugs', has historically been a means of oppressing minority groups in the USA. Jareki argues that currently the harsh and criminalising drug policy is economically driven and has a profound impact that affects all working-class groups; he suggests that the powerful economic bastion driving this is the privatised prison system.[25]

There have now been moves in two US states to decriminalise the possession of small amounts of cannabis and in 11 states it can be possessed for medical reasons; the patterns in the US may therefore be slowly changing or becoming more mixed. Other countries that take a hard line approach to drug use are Japan and Sweden. Because of consistent European monitoring it is possible to compare approaches and their effects and the results suggest that hard line approaches have negative health outcomes for drug users, with high levels of drug deaths and injecting use (*The Observer*, 23 May 2013).

Additionally, as noted above, a more tolerant or lenient approach has been pursued in Switzerland and the Czech Republic with regard to possession of small amounts of drugs and there has been no evidence that consumption has increased to any significant extent, nor has 'the roof fallen in' (UKDPC 2012: 120). Trautmann et al. (2013) writing about a sweep of research looking at different aspects of the European drug market have considered the recent Dutch move to tighten their restrictions on cannabis use within coffee shops in response to what they saw as problematic side effects from tourism as the result of their more liberal policies. Although legislation was introduced to restrict access to the coffee shops by people other than Dutch nationals – 'the weed pass' – this has been rarely implemented other than a small pilot scheme in one area of the Netherlands where an increase in street dealing appeared to result from the implementation; subsequently the idea was abandoned.

Furthermore, Trautmann et al. (2013) say that the status quo since the late 1960s of condoned cannabis use and small amounts for personal possession had brought positive benefits, such as an effective separation of the cannabis market from the opiate and cocaine markets. Additionally, some of those campaigning against the weed pass highlighted to the

---

[25] Jarecki's film won the Grand Jury Prize at the Sundance Film Festival 2012 and was also shown in the UK at that festival in 2012. You can read about it on the internet. The film is interesting to watch and an accessible introduction to some of the debates and issues about the interface between economic interests, discrimination and oppression and drug use policies.

government the potential for negative economic impact, both in terms of coffee shops closing and a subsequent reduction in tax revenue as the result of less potential trade.

In Portugal they went a step further and decided to decriminalise or depenalise the possession of small amounts of all drugs in 2001; the drugs themselves remain illegal, however, and thus the policy rather cleverly sought to 'get round' the international agreements to which Portugal is a signatory and which they acknowledge. It was also accompanied by a significant increase in the availability of drug treatment and use of harm reduction methods (*The Observer*, 23 May 2013). In Portugal, therefore, you can now possess without prosecution:

> *One gram of heroin, two grams of cocaine, 25 grams of marijuana leaves or five grams of hashish: These are the drug quantities one can legally purchase and possess in Portugal, carrying them through the streets of Lisbon in a pants pocket, say, without fear of repercussion. MDMA – the active ingredient in ecstasy – and amphetamines – including speed and meth – can also be possessed in amounts up to one gram. That's roughly enough of each of these drugs to last 10 days. These are the amounts listed in a table appended to Portugal's Law 30/2000.*
> (*Der Spiegel*, 27 March 2013)

The person leading this experiment is a doctor called João Goulão who considers the experiment has been successful and was a way to stop a drugs/crime cycle, open, street-based drug use and an approach that was not working. Portugal's geographical position has meant it is often an entry point into Europe for drugs and this too brought special problems (EMCDDA 2011). As the EMCDDA (2011) and UKDPC (2012) note there is some contention about the actual impact of the experiment but in Portugal the 'sky has not fallen in' as a result of decriminalisation. In general the EMCDDA (2011) report that while the strategy has not demonstrated significant results in terms of impact on problematic heroin use there have been other benefits and few negative impacts; thus Portugal has, and continues to have, a low level of drug trying and drug taking in comparison with other countries in Europe and its nearest neighbour, Spain.

Epidemiological models for calculating drug use, trying, prevalence, production, sales and supply are complex and different approaches, methods and statistical tests can be utilised. This can lead to arguments about the definitive 'results'; furthermore the impact of drug strategies takes time to assess. The USA has been a vociferous opponent of the move by Portugal and thus US coverage of the experiment has been more negative than others. However, despite initial opposition from the UN the approach of the USA has softened and they have now given tacit acceptance.

Portugal had, and continues to have, some of the lowest rates of drug use in Europe, except in the area of problematic heroin use, which the policy change sought to target. Heroin use was traditionally high with other negative health and social effects such as street-based drug dealing and use, IV use and high levels of drug-related deaths and HIV infections. Decriminalisation has positively impacted these effects and led to increased access to treatment, falling HIV rates and lowered levels of open or street drug use; there have been a range of other benefits including reductions in acquisitive crime and very low levels of recidivism among drug users (less than 8 per cent) (*Der Spiegel*, 27 March 2013; *Guardian* 2013; UKDPC 2012; Domosławski 2011). Additionally, there is a consensus that overall there have been few negative impacts.

The EMCDDA notes that the move by the Portuguese appears to have been in line with that of other governments, which has been towards a strategic approach to drug use through the creation of policy; an acceptance of harm reduction approaches; an increasing integration of licit and illicit drugs in the strategic response; and perhaps more controversially, a greater consideration of the health effects on the drug user (and a move away from consideration of the drug user as criminal).

However, there have been unintended or unforeseen effects. Thus, there is a requirement that if a person is stopped by the police and found in possession of a drug they must be referred to a panel, which assesses and decides on the necessity (or not) of intervention. What has been found is that this has disproportionately impacted on the young and the poor (Domosławski 2011) because they are the main targets of police intervention and stop and search; were this to be undertaken in the UK it is probable that we would see a disproportionate impact on the young, the poor and BME communities, because of the enduring disproportionate impact of stop and search policies within the UK (UKDPC 2012); it also offers a further warning of where the criminalisation of Khat use in the UK in 2013 may lead. The possibilities for structural factors to interact with policy are highlighted and the enduring aspects of oppressive behaviour and its negative impacts further exposed.

Harm reduction: toleration by another name?

Harm reduction remains contentious because it blurs the boundaries between what is acceptable and what is not; at the least it appears to tolerate or accommodate drug use. In this way what is or is not socially acceptable becomes in part a test of the normalisation or neutralisation theories of drug use within the wider community.

As we have seen, harm reduction measures, such as the provision of clean injecting equipment in the 1980s, proved incredibly successful as a weapon against HIV and blood-borne virus transmission. As drug use and users change, however, so new harm reduction measures also need to develop. In the 1990s there were debates about the provision of 'cool down' rooms and free drinking water in clubs because of the side effects of dance drug use such as ecstasy, which raised the body temperature, blood pressure and heart rate (DrugScope 2013). There are also current debates about the provision of safe injecting rooms and whether they reduce drug-related deaths; within the UK Brighton has considered introducing them, but their use has been more widespread in parts of Europe, such as Switzerland and Denmark. The debate in the UK has fractured in a way common in harm reduction debates, and coverage in *The Observer* (5 May 2013) contrasts sharply with commentary by Rod Liddle in the *Sunday Times* (21 April 2013). These sorts of debates help to highlight that drug use and intoxication, the toleration or acceptance of drug use/intoxication, and the limits within given societies and cultures were, and remain, varied.

Harm reduction measures target a variety of intoxicants, illicit and licit. They vary from needle exchange, drug consumption/injecting rooms, prescription heroin, 'free' water and 'cool down' rooms, licensing laws and the training and responsibilities of door staff at public venues. What they have in common is that they suggest that the use of intoxicants is not a moral matter, but a behaviour whose risks can be ameliorated – like wearing a seatbelt when driving. For some, this position in itself is not acceptable,[26] but for many it makes sense. Drug policies such as those implemented in the Netherlands since the late 1960s and more recently Portugal, have sought to divorce or limit the impact of moral judgements on criminal justice policy (particularly in relation to creating a separation between the markets selling 'soft' and 'hard' drugs – although this of course is also forming a judgement). Drug use in countries pursuing more liberal policies such as the Netherlands is no higher than in countries that have pursued a more prohibitionist stance such as the UK (Trautmann et al. 2013).

All of the above serves to highlight the complexities in this area, the ability for moral judgements, stereotypes and discrimination to impact on the views we take, the assessments we make and the judgements we form. It is important as a policy-maker or practitioner in this area that you are clear about your own views and reflective enough to ensure they do not impact on your practice causing you to be oppressive.

EXERCISE

Undertake an internet search on 'harm reduction' and another on drug consumption rooms or safe injecting rooms. Choose a number of articles that come from different perspectives and read them. Construct a mind map – show opinions/evidence in favour; opinions/evidence against; your view and why.

---

[26] For example see the comments of columnist Melanie Philips on *Question Time*, 20 June 2013, BBC1. She is opposed to harm minimisation, which she portrays as symptomatic of a failure to enforce drugs laws. In *The Spectator*, 27 May 2008, the UKDPC responded to what they considered had been erroneous allegations which she made against them in her *Spectator* Blog in the same month and year.

5 Why do people think that substance use is a problem?

Introduction

As we have seen in the previous chapters, people across the world and across time have considered that there are problematic effects associated with substance use. Those problematic effects are considered to be those that affect the individual substance user and those that affect those around them, be they family, peers and friendship networks, those who live near them, work with them or need to treat them for the health or other effects of intoxication. In addition there are the wider social effects of substance use, be it in the provision of licensing or the question of whose views and experiences should prevail; these sorts of arguments are currently and have been recently rehearsed in relation to alcohol licensing in the UK, the Police Reform Act (2011) and in the Alcohol Strategy (2012), discussed in Chapters 3 and 4. Additionally there are the effects of illegal or illicit drug trade, which are local, national and international and can have severe social and economic consequences such as those witnessed in some countries in South America and these are also discussed in Chapter 4. For those who argue for decriminalisation this is one of their key contentions – that the illegality of the trade leads to many of the negative effects associated with organised crime (see Transform Drug Policy Foundation in the UK[1]).

In this chapter we will draw on epidemiological studies regarding prevalence to understand more about the scale of the issue. We will also look at some research findings that have considered the impact of substance use on particular groups – for example children and young people, women, BME groups and older people – and the impact of substance use on mental health and terms such as 'dual diagnosis'. We will think about how difficult it can be for different groups of service users and their families to discuss or report the effects or scope of the substance use and how effective engagement can help to overcome these concerns.

[1] www.tdpf.org.uk

The intention is to enable those studying in this area or working in generic practice within social work, social care, the CJS, YJS, psychological services and healthcare, such as health visitors and school and district nurses, to be aware of the key issues regarding substance misuse and how this awareness can help them in their practice/ forthcoming practice.

The exploration of research findings in this chapter will enable the reader to think about the generic skills needed for assessment and intervention (for example communication skills) which can be employed to engage in generic practice with substance use/users.

LEARNING OUTCOMES

By the end of this chapter you should be able to:

» *Demonstrate your critical understanding of the research findings about prevalence within the UK and Europe regarding drug and alcohol.*

» *Critically evaluate the key debates about prevalence.*

» *Demonstrate your critical understanding and reflection of the impact of drug and alcohol use on particular groups of people.*

Research and substance use

Research concerned with prevalence of substance use is largely epidemiological, statistical and on occasions complex; in order to be able to interrogate it you need to be able to understand the methods used and the reasoning for choosing certain approaches and statistical tests. The evidence we discuss below with regard to prevalence has come from reputable sources subject to much consideration and debate and generally considered to be reliable and accurate; the reader can also source the studies and immerse themself in the statistical explanations and realities as the sources are given and the EMCDDA website is extremely helpful in providing access to detailed studies of prevalence across Europe.[2]

Other research around substance use takes a variety of approaches; some is quantitative, some qualitative and many studies draw on mixed methods – that is the combining of quantitative and qualitative methods. The importance of the methodological approach is that it is relevant to the question being asked – if you want to understand what the process of treatment was like or what it 'felt' like to live as a problematic drug user or receive a particular type of intervention then you would expect to read a qualitative study – one perhaps drawing on in-depth interviews or ethnographic methods. If, however, you want to know the impact or outcomes of certain inputs, for example what happens if you give all known injecting drug users in your area free, clean and easily accessible injecting equipment you would expect to see a quantitative methodology. What you might see, however, is a mixed method study which allows you to consider the impact and outcomes in terms of take up of the service, the

---

[2] For example: www.emcdda.europa.eu/publications/annual-report/2012

incidence of blood-borne disease and drug-related deaths, but you might also see interviews with the IV drug users to ascertain how accessible was the service, etc. Therefore when reading research in this area (as in general) ask yourself, do the methods chosen enable the question to be answered?

There are numerous studies of prevalence of drug use in particular in the UK and most of these post-date the first drug strategy, TDT 1995; thus data usually relate to the recent past. There was a real issue in the late 1980s and early 1990s about understanding how wide-spread the problem of drug use was. As we have discussed, drug issues and treatment were largely a 'Cinderella' area in health in the early 1990s and those who were concerned about what they saw as a changing pattern of drug use with criminal justice impacts felt they had little opportunity to understand or investigate it. The effect of these tensions was real and it was not a purely academic or semantic debate; for example if one does not know what is being used, how much, by whom, when and under what circumstances with any level of cer-tainty, you cannot plan for services, treatment or anticipate impacts. An indication of what the penal/medical tensions meant in practice was given by Joy Mott, who, speaking from a Home Office research perspective said that during the 1970s and 1980s:

> the Home Office could not fund research into treatment ...Then there is the question
> of epidemiology; that seemed to belong to the Dept of Health but it ended up with
> the Home Office putting questions on drug misuse into the British Crime Survey.
> (Mott 2000: 336)

Thus, tensions and debates about who had the 'right' to deal with drugs issues and how those varying perspectives could be debated, integrated and brought to bear, had a dir-ect impact on policy, service delivery, law, and the ability to 'know' what was happening through research. These were the days before 'joined-up government' and they serve as a reminder of the very discrete ways in which the big institutions of state operated. Moreover, the introduction of the questions on the British Crime Survey (BCS) turned out to be very useful regarding the question of drug trying and its wider impacts and these have continued although they have become more sophisticated over time. The survey has now changed its name to become the Crime Survey of England and Wales (CSEW).

Organisations such as the DATs, DPI, DPAS and then the NTA, in response to the various gov-ernment strategies, have since the mid-1990s also increased the amount that we now 'know' about drug use, drug trying and other health, criminal justice and social effects. Equally, Europe also now requires the collection and collation of large amounts of epidemiological data and commissions other types of research, including in-depth qualitative studies.

The interesting thing about substance use is that it is an ever changing scene and there-fore this book will concentrate on ensuring an understanding of key and ongoing issues and debates, as well as presenting some 'headline' figures and issues with which policy-makers are currently grappling. Once again the best place to follow in detail the current patterns of use and supply is through the government and EMCDDA websites.

The EMCDDA (2012a) report highlights concerns about the impact of the economic and financial downturn in Europe and its potential to impact drug use. It suggests that countries need to think clearly about the costs and benefits of drug treatment services and identifies six countries in Europe that have made recent cuts to specified drug budgets; these include the UK with a 5 per cent drop in expenditure in 2010/11. There is also what appears an underlying, though unspoken, worry about the possible structural impact of unemployment and disaffection, which could result in a pattern of drug use more similar to the late 1970s and 1980s.

The report details a changing pattern of cannabis supply which is now often locally grown and supplied, rather than imported – this affects the product, which may vary considerably across Europe (EMCDDA 2012a). The involvement of organised crime and the development of sophisticated growing, harvesting and yield technologies causes some concern for policy-makers who seek to find ways to cope with the changing pattern of supply. How they respond to this is clearly important because cannabis remains the most popular illicit substance in terms of trying and continued use. Because of the locally produced nature of cannabis across Europe it has become a diverse product with differential properties, and as a result it is more difficult to generalise about effects.

The EMCDDA (2012a) also highlight that cocaine and heroin continue to be relevant to the majority of drug-associated harms in terms of health and criminal justice outcomes. The EMCDDA (2012a: 73) defines problem drug use as *injecting drug use or long duration or regular use of opioids, cocaine or amphetamines*. Thus cocaine and heroin are both speci-fied drugs and both are used on occasions intravenously; the prevalence of their use is there-fore also relevant to both potential or actual problematic use and drug-related harms.

In terms of prevalence there can be wide variations across Europe in terms of drug taking and drug trying, but the combined data suggest that it remains a minority activity and that of those adults who have ever used a drug 23.7 per cent of Europeans have tried cannabis, 4.6 per cent cocaine, 3.4 per cent ecstasy and 3.8 per cent amphetamines. Opiod (for example heroin) use remains very low – less than 1 per cent of 1.4 million adults across Europe have ever tried it; the negative harms associated with opiod use, however, remain significant, accounting for 50 per cent of all requests for treatment and 75 per cent of drug-related deaths of which 4 per cent in Europe are drug induced (EMCDDA 2012a: 17).

Prevalence of use in the UK

The use of substances in the UK remains towards the higher end of the spectrum across Europe despite recent and sustained falls. The EMCDDA studies (2102a, 2012c) on the UK report higher 'ever' usage of cannabis than for other European countries; it also highlights the more complex picture now with Northern Ireland and Scotland reporting separately, which affects the comparable rates, etc. and Northern Ireland adopting a different method of 'counting' prevalence, which is the same as that used in some other European countries (see EMCDDA reports for more detail[3]).

Interestingly, the UKDPC (2012: 77) report graphically demonstrated that there is a close relationship between levels of income distribution and prevalence of substance use, provid-ing further evidence that socio-economic factors are in some way related (at the very least) to substance use. Additionally, the UKDPC highlight that cultural factors may also play a role –for example the encouragement of 'hedonism' and the prevalence of the use of alcohol.

---

[3] www.emcdda.europa.eu/publications/country-overviews/uk 2013

What is reported is that, for those aged 16–59 living in England and Wales in 2011/12 36.5 per cent had ever tried any illicit drug (lifetime prevalence rates). For particular drugs 'ever' trying was:

- cannabis 31 per cent;
- amphetamines 11.5 per cent;
- cocaine 9.6 per cent;
- ecstasy 8.6 per cent;
- LSD 5.3 per cent.

For those who had used a drug in 2011/12 the prevalence was:

- cannabis use 6.9 per cent (maintaining a steady decline since 2003/04, from 10.8 per cent) and stabilisation since 2009/10. Current cannabis use was more prevalent among 16- to 24-year-olds than among older respondents. But those who continued cannabis use as they grew older more frequently reported daily or almost daily use of the substance. This is relevant therefore for those practising with older cannabis users.

- Cocaine use has also decreased, but because of increases in 2008/9 it remains the second most frequently used drug.

- Amphetamine use has also continued to decrease and this pattern has been consistent since 2003.

- 1.1 per cent of respondents used mephedrone in the last 12 months, a decrease from 1.4 per cent in 2010/11. Among 16- to 24-year-olds mephedrone use decreased from 4.4 per cent in 2010/11 to 3.3 per cent in 2011/12.

The patterns of use in Scotland and Northern Ireland are slightly lower for having 'ever' used a drug than for England and Wales, sitting at just under one-third; thus for 2010/11:

- 29.2 per cent of those aged 16–64 in Scotland;
- 27.3 per cent in Northern Ireland, based on 2010/11.

There are also a number of school surveys across the UK, with that in England undertaken since 1998. For details of each survey please consult the EMCDDA website but essentially what was shown was declining numbers of drug trying and taking, such that:

> The school age population study in England confirms a long-term declining trend in lifetime prevalence of cannabis use among 15-year-olds from 37% in 2003 to 21% in 2011.

This finding was further validated by data from other studies in the UK:

> latest HBSC results for 2010 also indicate a decline in lifetime cannabis prevalence rates among 15-year-olds from 36% in 1998 to 22% in Wales, and from 37% in 2002 to 19% in Scotland.

The studies above are based mainly on self-reported behaviour, which is not without its drawbacks – for example we know that people often minimise the amount of alcohol they drink.

However, the falls shown are similar to those shown in previous surveys so it is unlikely that they are inaccurate in terms of in trying and use – but overall, all of the surveys may under-estimate how much each person has used.

In other recent surveys of the use of serious or 'harder' drugs we have also seen a decline in use with a national fall in the prevalence of opiate and/or crack cocaine use between 2009/10 and 2010/11 and a statistically significant decrease in the levels of crack cocaine use, alongside a significant decrease in injecting prevalence rates (Hay et al. 2011: 2). There *were also statistically significant decreases in the prevalence of opiate and/or crack cocaine use within the 15 to 24 and 25–34 age groups* and *the prevalence of drug injecting has also significantly decreased* (Hay et al. 2011: 19). Although there was an increase in the number of opiate and/or crack cocaine users in the older 35 to 64 age group it is considered that this group may comprise older users whose drug use dates from the 1980s and 1990s and who have now progressed into treatment and/or 'moved up' the age categories; there is no real concern therefore that drug use within this group in itself has increased. This is an area directly relevant to practice and practitioners and also of significance to district nurses, who need to be aware that there may be a greater likelihood of use and/or dependent opiate or crack cocaine use in the over 35 population with whom they work, than among young people.

Drug supply as business

There are sustained attempts by governments, policy-makers and researchers to under-stand the manufacture and supply of illicit drugs, which because of its illegal nature is cov-ert, hidden and associated with criminal activity. The production, supply and distribution of drugs is not the principal focus here but does warrant a brief mention, in part because of its undoubted relevance, but also because many who have worked in drug production and supply will come into contact with those working within the health, social care and criminal justice systems. There are also anecdotal suggestions from practice and concerns reported in the media that the trafficking of children to work on cannabis production means that these young people are erroneously being brought into the CJS on occasions, or that when they become known to social services they are often 'lost' back to the organised criminal gangs; the effect is that the children and young people are not being assisted and supported (*Sunday Times*, 25 August 2013). As a reader of this book you are urged again to think about any possible stereotypes you might have and to ensure that you consider the extreme experi-ences and circumstances it is suggested some young people who have been made to work in this area have been through.

There are many interesting studies by people such as Dunlap (1995) and Bourgois (2003) both from the USA, which have retained a strong tradition of the use of ethnographic meth-ods in understanding drug use and exploring drug supply. Most studies focus in particular at a grass-roots level because gaining access to people higher up the supply chain is difficult. Recent research by Trautmann et al. (2013) for the EU used a different methodology that enabled them to study illegal markets by looking at case studies of 33 failed incidents of cocaine smuggling-related transactions in the Netherlands. They found that conflict reso-lution between parties was in the majority of incidents dealt with much as it would be in legal markets, thus through resolution:

The data show that in most instances the Ringleader follows routines perhaps not very different from those in legitimate organizations, investigating whether the balance of evidence favours an interpretation of bad luck or underling incompetence as opposed to an effort to defraud.

(Trautmann et al. 2013: 32)

They also concluded that the potential for conflict and resultant use of violence might be higher than in traditional business settings because risk was also greater with the illegality of the trade – thus written contracts, negotiations and other legalised forms of trust could not be resorted to.

This finding is congruent with Dunlap's (1995) findings in her smaller scale but more detailed ethnographic study and in some ways both go towards challenging the stereotypes of the necessarily violent way in which drug production and supply is managed.

Trautmann et al. (2013) also looked at the way *criminal organisations operate as 'polymorphous criminal networks', responding to changes in their markets by looking for alternative – licit and illicit – ways to secure their position and income.* As a result they proposed a *new framework for a better understanding of the relationships between the diverse activities undertaken by internationally operating criminal networks in particular those involved in illicit drug trafficking* (Trautmann et al. 2013: 31).[4]

Working with substance users

Key messages from research are that treatment works; however, recovery may take a long time (for example Marsh and Cao 2005). Numerous studies consistently demonstrate that there is a reduction in harms associated with substance use when a user maintains contact with a treatment service and that this benefits those around them (within their family and within their community) and minimises the harms associated with drug use (NTA 2013; UKDPC 2012; Gossop et al. 2001; Marsh and Cao 2005). Within the treatment and policy world there is also increased focus on resiliency and in particular how resiliency might be developed and supported within individuals and families. Furthermore, it is suggested that there is a treatment effect such that it contributes to the levels of resilience and commitment to change which support controlled use or drug-free lives (EMCDDA 2012a; Marsh and Cao 2005). We will consider treatment approaches further and in more detail in Chapter 6; however, it is important to underline this issue when considering the impact that substance use may have directly or indirectly on specific groups of people within society.

Young people

Substance trying

The trend across Europe remains stable for drug use and drug trying among young people and this includes cannabis. The pattern that had been worrying governments and was outside of this trend was heavy, episodic drinking – 'binge drinking' – which was seen to be increasing and causing concern; Berridge (2007), however, notes that the same level of concern did not appear to have been given to other areas of increased alcohol consumption,

---

[4] Further insights into aspects of the EU illicit drugs market: Trautmann et al. 2013.

such as in the family and in the home. Despite concerns, the EMCDDA (2012a: 14) suggest that across Europe the 'binge' drinking trend appears to be slowing or diminishing. They also note that:

> countries that report high prevalence estimates for one substance, tend also to report relatively high estimates for other substances, both licit and illicit, thus high levels of recent use of alcohol and heavy episodic drinking are associated with the use of illicit drugs and inhalants.

The conclusion they draw is that this *supports prevention approaches that recognise the need to target both drugs and alcohol when working with young people* (EMCDDA 2012a: 14) and not therefore simply targeting messages about a particular substance or to a particular group. As many young people across Europe and all within the UK receive some form of drug education or prevention advice this is an important message and we will look further at this in the following chapter.[5] Other studies moreover indicate that while young people have shown increasing levels of 'knowledge' about drugs this in fact has amounted to knowing their names and not their effects (Wright and Pearl 2000). Wright and Pearl's study has implications for educational messages indicating a need to deliver content about the effects of drugs in a way which is intelligible. Otherwise, as it demonstrated, the media remains the principal source of information for young people (followed by friends and then talk in school) and as we know the media's portrayals can be inaccurate, overly focused on celebrity and death and stigmatising (UKDPC 2012).

In terms of prevalence, the findings about falling use are important because substance use trying in the adolescent phase indicates an increased likelihood to try other substances at a later stage. This is of course loosely related as the 'ever' trying categories for alcohol, tobacco and cannabis are much higher than for any other substance and we know that drug use is associated with regular smoking and recent drinking in young people – thus drug trying is not a 'stepping stone' to drug use as some have suggested, but does indicate a greater willingness to 'try' and to take risk – both of which indicate an increased probability that you might do so with regard to other things and/or substances. Additionally, for epidemiologists the pattern that develops in this group is of interest because it indicates possible patterns of 'trying' or use in the future and thus for policy-makers and practitioners it helps them to consider and plan for future treatment needs.

What we know more generally about prevalence and young people aged 11–15 in 2011 is the following:

- Drug trying and use increases with age – 23 per cent of 15-year-olds had ever tried a drug compared to 3 per cent of 11-year-olds.

- Gender and ethnicity make little difference to overall use – this is a change, especially regarding ethnicity, as previously being white had a been a risk factor and being from a BME group had been a protective factor.

---

[5] The scale of drug education and prevention advice that goes into schools across the UK is not, for example, mirrored in countries such as Germany; patterns within and across Europe vary considerably.

- There has been a decline in drug use with just 17 per cent ever having taken a drug (29 per cent in 2001).

- There has been a decline in those ever offered a drug – 29 per cent (42 per cent in 2001).

- Just 12 per cent had taken a drug in the last year and 6 per cent in the last month.

- The drugs young people try are cannabis (7.6 per cent) and/or glue, gas or other volatile substance (3.5 per cent). Less than 1 per cent of 11- to 15-year-olds had tried any other substance.

- Younger children sniff volatile substances and were more likely to report having 'felt no different' having done so (75 per cent); whereas 14- to 16-year-olds are more likely to have smoked cannabis and to report that they 'felt good' doing so (58 per cent).

- Feeling good or experiencing no difference is important to subsequent use with 41 per cent of those who said they felt good the first time they took drugs doing so on six or more occasions; whereas those who felt no difference or who felt bad were unlikely to use again (just 10 per cent and 7 per cent respectively).

- The minority use drugs with any frequency – just over a one-third (35 per cent) who had used drugs previously had done so in the last month, which is equivalent to just 3 per cent of 11- to 15-year-olds in total.

- Around one-third (29 per cent) of those who had ever taken drugs had only done so once.

- Of those who had ever taken drugs 58 per cent said they wanted to stop now or in the future, but just 4 per cent thought they needed help or treatment.

- The majority of young people who had been offered a drug had refused at least once (75 per cent); their reasons for doing so included: *I just didn't want to take them*; *I think taking drugs is wrong*; *I thought they were dangerous* and *I didn't want to get addicted*.
(Source: Health and Social Care Information Centre, 2011)

Working with young people

The implications for practice from the above findings are that drug use among those under 15 is a minority activity and that at most it may be drug trying or infrequent use and that it is almost never anything more than cannabis, and among younger people, volatile substances. Where a different picture is presented of ongoing or frequent use or the use of 'harder' substances such as Class A drugs it would be wise to undertake an initial assessment or refer the young person for further assessment.

Working with young people around the issues of substance use is affected by some additional legislation (including the Children Act 2004 as previously discussed) and different considerations, for example:

- *Drugs: Protecting Families and Communities* (Home Office 2008) integrated substance use services into mainstream children's services in order to make them more child friendly and accessible. It also sought to strengthen the role of schools in identifying problems and improving drug education delivered in school.

- The *Youth Alcohol Action Plan* (DCSF et al. 2008) outlined the government's response to problematic drinking among young people and aimed to influence attitudes to alcohol and patterns of drinking, particularly binge drinking.

- *Working Together to Safeguard Children* (DCSF 2010) and *Every Child Matters* (Department of Education 2004) both apply although they exist within a changing social care landscape and have been the subject of change. There is now less prescription from the centre and a greater focus on localities making local decisions. However, there is a requirement to publish in full Serious Case Reviews, an expectation that a more systematic methodology will be applied to reviews within social services and an enhanced focus on individual, professional responsibility and accountability across all professional groups within health and social care settings. A practitioner therefore should be aware of local arrangements and expectations and ensure that they exercised their professional judgement in accordance with their professional group's expectations and ethics, for example British Association of Social Work (BASW), Health and Care Professions Council (HCPC), etc.

- *Positive for Youth* (HM Government 2012) is an overall cross-government strategy aimed at young people. It shows congruence with preceding strategies (such as drug strategies and those for youth offending) in being cross-government. It suggests that it wishes to move away from negative stereotypes of young people and towards more positive portrayal and engagement; however, there has appeared to be little impact in practice and many cuts have in fact settled upon and impacted the young, for example cuts to library and sports facilities, cuts to outreach and youth services, etc. The NSPCC (2009) note that despite government rhetoric the overall approach to young people remains a focus on the risk that they *pose* rather than the risks that they *face.*

The overall focus in the guidance is to minimise harm(s) to young people and to ensure a clear identification of those harms or potential harms (NTA 2007). Practitioners must remember that young people aged under 16 years are usually dependent and may be subject to other legal restrictions, for example the use of alcohol if under the age of 18 years. They may have parents, carers or guardians who may wish to be involved in assessments or feel that they should be informed about substance use, etc.; it is important therefore practitioners are quite clear what the local protocols, expectations and agreements are, for example, confidentiality and disclosure regarding young people.[6]

Furthermore, research by Leavey et al. (2011) has shown that young people evidenced *a worrying lack of confidence and trust* in family doctors (GPs) and other professionals when seeking help. Help-seeking was mediated by factors relevant to adults, for example social class, but there was also a clear lack of trust shown by young people combined with perceptions that one sought help from GPs for physical problems not mental health ones (Leavey et al. 2011). The authors raised concerns that depression was significantly under-diagnosed among young people and that there was a perceived insensitivity to young people's concerns (Leavey et al. 2011); they suggested that generic practitioners such as GPs should get to know young people better when they were well and to form relationships of trust – this has direct relevance for generic practitioners and substance use.

---

[6] For example, see Fraser Guidelines and Gillick Competency NSPCC 2012: www.nspcc.org.uk/inform/research/questions/gillick_wda61289.html

Risks for young people

Recent enquiries, reviews and court cases have highlighted the risks to some young people from unscrupulous and abusive adults who use substances both to entice young people into relationships and then use those substances to control them.[7] There have been examples of this sort of behaviour over many years and it has occurred in previous Serious Case Reviews, for example Aliyah Ismail (Fox and Arnull 2013), but the recent furore over and considerable press coverage of the sexual exploitation of girls in particular has strongly featured the integrated use of substances as a hook and a tie and brought such considerations more forcefully to the fore in generic practice. As a result, new guidance has been issued and this also draws out the strong relationship that is known to exist between previous experiences of victimisation and more general delinquency (Fox and Arnull 2013). What the Consultation on the Interim Guidance on Prosecuting Cases of Child Sexual Abuse issued by the Director of Public Prosecutions on 11 June 2013 says is as follows:

> *Typical vulnerabilities in children prior to abuse:*
> * *living in a chaotic or dysfunctional household (including parental substance use, domestic violence, parental mental health issues, parental criminality);*
> * *history of abuse (including familial child sexual abuse, risk of forced marriage, risk of 'honour'-based violence, physical and emotional abuse and neglect);*
> * *recent bereavement or loss;*
> * *gang association either through relatives, peers or intimate relationships (in cases of gang associated CSE only);*
> * *attending school with young people who are sexually exploited;*
> * *learning disabilities;*
> * *unsure about their sexual orientation or unable to disclose sexual orientation to their families;*
> * *friends with young people who are sexually exploited;*
> * *homeless;*
> * *lacking friends from the same age group;*
> * *living in a gang neighbourhood;*
> * *living in residential care;*
> * *living in hostel, bed and breakfast accommodation or a foyer;*
> * *low self-esteem or self-confidence;*
> * *young carer.*

The breadth of these risk factors is like the other research in this area: it 'captures' so many more people than are affected or likely to be affected; it also includes those who are already vulnerable, victimised and often poor or living in socially deprived areas. However, they do serve to highlight the importance for generic practitioners to be aware of risk factors and be able to explore critically, reflectively and analytically what they see before them and not simply respond to the immediate issue, or behaviour. We know this occurred with the young women in Rochdale and in the case of Aliyah Ismail all of whom were on occasions dismissed

---

[7] Goodman (2007: 70) discusses some of the earlier research in this area for example by Cusick, Martin and May (2003) and 'trapping' factors including 'prostitution' before the age of 13; the terminology has now changed in this area but Cusick et al.'s findings have subsequently been substantiated by recent events.

or ignored, often because young people experiencing extreme circumstances can be diffi-cult to engage (Fox and Arnull 2013: 51). Thus, when undertaking assessments with young people (and adults) many of whom will have experienced other health and social care inter-ventions in the past and have experienced a range of psychosocial, environmental, medical and structural problems and difficulties, you should be looking at the whole picture, not a part. Again the new guidance suggests important factors regarding child sexual exploitation and victimisation may include:

> *The following signs and behaviour are generally seen in children who are already being sexually exploited:*
> * *missing from home or care;*
> * *physical injuries;*
> * *drug or alcohol misuse;*
> * *involvement in offending;*
> * *repeat sexually-transmitted infections, pregnancy and terminations;*
> * *absent from school;*
> * *change in physical appearance;*
> * *evidence of sexual bullying and/or vulnerability through the internet and/or social networking sites;*
> * *estranged from their family;*
> * *receipt of gifts from unknown sources;*
> * *recruiting others into exploitative situations;*
> * *poor mental health;*
> * *self-harm;*
> * *thoughts of or attempts at suicide.*
>
> (DPP 11 June 2013)

Areas of potential problematic factors therefore include substance use by parents and fam-ilies or by the child or young person themselves. As we have seen and shall discuss in more detail below, dependent or problematic substance use by a young person is very rare, but there are indicative factors that increase the probability that this might occur or be occurring. This highlights the importance of being able to see, understand and consider the relevance of generic risk factors and then relate those to the actual person(s) or family. If a practitioner finds a cluster of behaviours or areas of concern for a young person they should consider undertaking an open, accurate, generic comprehensive assessment at an early stage as this may be important in indicating risk factors and identifying areas of resilience, which may be important in supporting and enabling the young person in the future. Be prepared to find and accept that there is no problem, but where dependent or problematic use is indicated specialist advice and support or referral should be sought.

Young people give their own accounts for why they choose to take drugs and other sub-stances and there is a considerable body of research that has looked at what influences the likelihood that a young person will take drugs or other substances. What is consistently drawn out is a range of factors with which generic practitioners will already be familiar (Fox and Arnull 2013). As Fox and Arnull (2013: 40) discuss, it is important for practitioners to engage with young people on the understanding that during adolescence, delinquency is *a common, transitional, developmental phase between childhood and adulthood* and this is *a helpful way to balance, reflect upon and consider the behaviour at hand.* Many young people engage in delinquent behaviour(s) at some point and most come to no harm and leave it behind them (Fox and Arnull 2013; Smith et al. 2001). Furthermore in countries where substance use is more common (such as the UK) those who are low risk substance users may be more likely to been seen by generic services, but may not go on to develop problems, difficulties or dependencies (EMCDDA 2012a; UKDPC 2012). Additionally, Young and West's (2010) findings regarding the influence of 'good values' on health behaviour found there was no evidence *that holding certain 'pro-social' or 'good' values substantively protects against later substance use* and they challenged assumptions that values-based education would have this effect. They suggested that if government wanted to promote 'values-based' education it could do so, but this was not a public health issue per se. We will discuss further universal educational programmes as a prevention strategy in the following chapter; what is worth noting, however, is that the area is complex with educational inputs trying to 'hit' numerous variables with significant other inputs and effects. Furthermore, the findings of Young and West (2010) suggest that using substances might no longer be perceived as taking a non-pro-social stance – which would be interesting in itself.

Overall, the indicators are that it is important not to assume that something is, or will become, problematic, even if contact with a service is made. Delinquency includes a range of behaviours, which include substance trying and use – common risk and protective factors and resiliency are therefore all applicable. Important factors for substance use, and especially problematic use, appear to include how able the young person is to cope with loss, difficulties and trauma and whether they look for substances to provide mediation or alleviation. Key factors related to substance use are:

*   boredom;
*   social situations;
*   sensation seeking;
*   good fun;
*   lack of work or opportunity;
*   escaping family problems;
*   something your family does;
*   lack of strong parental attachment/involvement;
*   aggressiveness;
*   impulsivity;
*   mental health problems;
*   offending;
*   truanting or exclusion from school;
*   in care/accommodated by the LA;
*   becoming engaged in sex work or becoming sexually exploited;
*   being involved with or part of a gang.

Young people who are resilient and have other social characteristics that make it unlikely that substance use will become harmful to them are, for example, those who have a good relationship with their parents and whose parents are able to apply appropriate boundaries and who know where the young person is (Fox and Arnull 2013; Rosenkranz et al. 2012; Smith et al. 2001).

Young people can be at greater risk of harm as the result of drug trying and use because the experience is new to them and so they have less experience and in general try substances with others who are inexperienced. This reasoning formed the background to my submission to Drinkaware in which I discussed issues about young people's access to a more controlled drinking environment, such as a pub, when beginning to drink alcohol. For example, evidence indicates that adverts expose young people to social models of drinking but they are in fact more likely to be influenced by the behaviour of their peers, parents and other adults with whom they have a close relationship, rather than people they do not know nor care about (Martino et al. 2006; Bremner et al. 2011); this is subtly but importantly different from what they think they 'know' about substances and where they 'learn' this (Wright and Pearl 2000). In a country therefore with relatively high levels of 'ever' trying and repeated use of alcohol, it seems most appropriate that young people are exposed to pro-social models of controlled alcohol use; this is more likely in a controlled social environment such as a pub, than a park. If we also want to decrease the risks of harm we would want to limit how often young people drink alone or in environments that may also pose greater risk, and therefore prevention strategies would need to promote pro-social, controlled drinking environments – essentially this is employing harm minimisation strategies more commonly associated with drug use and the provision of water and 'cool down' rooms, etc.

For young people the adolescent phase is about lots of physical, emotional and psychological change as well as many social, educational and other pressures; failing or becoming involved in problematic or harmful behaviours can occur around this time and for some young people it can be the start of a lifetime of difficulties (Fox and Arnull 2013; Smith et al. 2001). There is evidence that most young people are not very different from one another in terms of the things they do (Smith et al. 2001) but that the effects can be differential. Thus social class and poverty are mediating factors that make it more likely that you will be arrested when other factors are held constant; as will the experience of being taken into care. Ethnicity used to have a differential effect on drug trying and use but this appears to have changed in recent times; as has gender (Health and Social Care Information Centre 2011).

There is some emerging evidence, however, that programmes that are educational and generic but targeted at groups already involved in other forms of delinquency do show a treatment effect. Thus, a study by Kim and Leve (2011) using an RCT design to evaluate the efficacy of an intervention to reduce substance use and delinquency among a group of girls in foster care found that at a 36-month follow-up period there was a statistically significant lower level of substance use among the treatment group. They concluded that this highlighted *the importance of providing preventative intervention services*[8] and noted that

---

[8] The findings for more general delinquency/offending showed a treatment effect but not one that was statistically significant; this would be in line with other research on delinquency and girls which indicates the importance of targeted criminogenic programmes; see Arnull and Eagle 2009.

the positive effects appeared related to increased pro-social behaviours which decreased *internalising and externalising symptoms* (Kim and Leve 2011: 740).

Additionally, Rosenkranz et al. (2012: 445) has suggested that there were positive effects of a *trauma-informed treatment approach* for young people with histories of psychological mal-treatment (emotional abuse or neglect) whom they found to be statistically more susceptible to develop substance use dependencies/problems than those who had other abuse histories. They suggested that treatment aimed at *enhancing adaptive coping skills, developing an adaptive sense of self and improving interpersonal relationship capacities* would help the young person with their substance dependency and also enable them to develop the skills they were missing because of the effects of psychological maltreatment or neglect as children or young people. This is an important finding as other research indicates that the most common and least noted and referred form of maltreatment is emotional abuse and neglect (Gilbert et al. 2009).

Gilbert et al. (2009) argue that there is a need for better initial assessment and referral by generic practitioners and this is congruent with the findings of Leavey et al. (2011). Generic practitioners are the most likely to come into contact with children who are being emotionally abused or neglected, but they are chronically under-referred. Gilbert et al. found this was because generic practitioners such as health and community-based practitioners, such as school nurses and paediatricians:

- lacked understanding about what constituted a reason for referral;

- were confused about whether another factor might account for the area giving them cause for concern;

- were worried about damaging their relationship with the parents/child.

Gilbert et al. (2009) argue that more training in this area is needed, alongside a greater use of validated assessment checklists at an early stage in order to highlight areas for concern and lead to a referral.[9] Furthermore, an enhanced, general acceptance about the importance of inter-disciplinary and shared responsibility for identifying the maltreatment of children and a move away from blaming and stigmatising parents and towards a supportive or investigative approach would be helpful. They note, however, that if more cases were identified children and family services might not be able to cope. Their recommendations have relevance for how issues of emotional neglect or maltreatment might be better recognised and engaged with by generic practitioners and perhaps as a result lead over time to improved outcomes for children and consequently fewer substance-dependent lives.

During adolescence young people's bodies and brains are still developing and thus the impacts of substances may differ or be felt more profoundly by them. They may also impair young people's functioning or help them to mask other symptoms or changes they are experiencing and with which they are uncomfortable. The well-known debate about the likelihood that cannabis use 'causes' mental health or psychotic symptoms has focused principally on

---

[9] Cox and Bentovim (2000) have put together for the DoH a whole range of validated questionnaires and scales that can be used for assessment: they can all be found at www.clusterweb.org.uk/UserFiles/CW/File/Policy/Childrens_Social_Services/CHIN/Policy_Procedure_and_Guidance/AF05_DoH_Family_Pack_Questionnaires_and_Scales_0907.pdf

the young, and the research evidence is at best unclear. What is indicated is that psychotic symptoms often onset in young people during adolescence and early adulthood and this is also a time when young people try new things and take risks. For those who are experiencing mental health issues such as psychosis or depression the use of cannabis may help to relieve or mask those symptoms and the interplay can therefore be considered to be 'confounding', making certainty about cause and effect difficult to ascertain. Fox et al. (2011) used a number of validated tools including a five factor structure to ask young people a number of questions related to differential motivations for cannabis use and found that *using cannabis to cope with negative affect had the strongest and most robust relationships with negative use-related consequences* (Fox et al. 2011: 498). For example, some young people indicated that they used cannabis *because it helps me when I am depressed or anxious* whereas others might choose another option *because it makes social gatherings more fun.* The importance of their findings for practice are that they are in line with other studies that indicate that it is important to assess the coping motive for cannabis use (and other substance use) as that is a potential predictor for negative effects.

In a systematic review conducted in 2007, however, Moore et al. stated that there was no evidence that cannabis use among young people contributed to depression, suicidal thoughts or anxiety but that there was a link between dosage and psychotic symptoms (ie high levels of use = more likely to have psychotic symptoms), which appeared to remain even when confounding factors were taken into account. They concluded therefore that:

> *The evidence is consistent with the view that cannabis increases risk of psychotic outcomes independently of confounding and transient intoxication effects ... [and thus] conclude that there is now sufficient evidence to warn young people that using cannabis could increase their risk of developing a psychotic illness later in life.*
>
> (Moore et al. 2007)

This was an important finding and one that contradicted an earlier systematic review also published in *The Lancet* in 2004 that had found cannabis use among young people to be associated with:

* lower educational attainment;
* increased reported use of other illicit drugs.

It did not find a relationship with psychological health problems or problematic behaviour, which the authors concluded were *explicable in terms of non-causal mechanisms* (Macleod et al. 2004). Arsenault et al. (2004) similarly concluded that there was no evidence that cannabis use caused psychosis but appeared to be *a component cause, part of a constellation of factors.*

What the evidence indicates overall therefore is that there is not a known or definitively proven link between cannabis use in adolescent years and psychosis. Thus, most young people who smoke cannabis will probably not suffer ill effects such as psychosis and there is no demonstrable link with depression, suicidal thoughts or anxiety although there is a suggestion that those who use cannabis to help themselves cope with problems will be more likely to suffer other negative effects associated with use. However, the risk of psychotic symptoms may be increased for some young people who smoke frequently or smoke a lot of cannabis. The implication for practice is therefore to be quite clear what the individual young person with whom you may be engaged is actually doing, what motivates their use (for example pleasure seeking or as a coping strategy) and how frequently they use; finally that once that assessment is completed they understand the possible risk their use might pose to themselves.

A well demonstrated area of risk for young people with regard to substance trying and use is parental conflict. This has been found to be a factor related to other forms of delinquency and across cultures. Within the UK a longitudinal prospective study, the Edinburgh Study (Smith et al. 2001) found this effect across all social groups and the recent enquiries regarding sexual exploitation have found young people who are distanced from their parents by force (because they are in LA care for example) or because of conflict, are most at risk of exploitation by unscrupulous adults (Cusick and Hickman 2005). In addition, an interesting study by Webber (2002) highlights the differential impact of culture, race and immigration and how these too can play a role. Her study in Australia with Vietnamese-Australian families also found conflict with parents/within the family to be a factor implicated in young people's propensity to take risks, which included drug trying and use. Of relevance to practitioners is the enduring importance of this aspect of family life during the adolescent phase. Webber found a strong degree of *agreement between the parent and youth cohorts about the nature of cross-generational conflict* (2002: 23) but the two groups attributed the cause of the conflict to different things:

*   parents blamed Australian lifestyle and culture;

*   young people blamed parental behaviour and *their parents' inability to embrace Western freedoms*.

Webber suggested that the practice implications for her research were to consider preventative work that aimed to assist parents and their children *to work out ways of managing the ensuing conflicts*, in particular where the issues arose from differential expectations about family, cultural values and parenting practices. The study has very real resonance for practice in the UK with families and young people, and is an important area for consideration where families have immigrated into the UK and/or where cultural values between generations are unshared or conflictual.

Finally, there is a growing body of evidence that links substance use among young people with group or gang behaviour. This is related both to the selling of drugs and to 'initiation' rites or ceremonies. The latter also appears to be affecting groups of young people involved in sports clubs in particular at universities where initiation ceremonies may involve consuming considerable quantities of alcohol regardless of physical size, gender, previous drinking experience and tolerance or other factors, which may be relevant to toleration of those quantities of alcohol (Wright, unpublished work[10]). The former may be more powerful at 'locking in' young people to ongoing forms of delinquent or substance using behaviour but the latter can expose some young people to harms, especially in the short term.

---

[10] Jane Wright unpublished and ongoing research 'The Impact of Alcohol on the Socialisation of Undergraduates into University'.

EXERCISE

Assessment exercise: draw on a case that includes a young person with whom you have been working, or who lives in a family with whom you are working, where there has been a question mark about possible substance use. Answer the following:[11]

1. Who is concerned about what and why?

2. What are the risks?

3. What are the positives/strengths?

4. Who should you contact/speak to?

5. What is your hypothesis about what is going on?

6. With whom and how can you verify or disprove the information you have/your hypothesis?

7. What are some possible outcomes?

8. What are the advantages of each outcome?

9. What are the disadvantages of each outcome?

Families and parents who are drug users

The greatest 'risks' and potential harms regarding substance use for children and young people are accessed via adults, eg risks:

*   posed by substance use of a parent or carer who has responsibility for them;

*   arising from being removed from the family home and going into care;

*   becoming disengaged from school;

*   involved in delinquency;

*   by an exploitative adult or abuser who gains access to them.

It is estimated that at least 60,000 children across Europe are living with parents who are illicit drug users who are in treatment and more children than that are estimated to be in contact with a drug-using parent who is not in treatment. There have been a number of European wide studies focused on families and substance-dependent parents (EMCDDA 2012b); it is important when considering these findings in the light of generic practice that the reader understands that the studies are referring to those with serious, dependent, problematic use. The findings suggest that those with illicit drug problems do not necessarily make 'bad' parents but are likely to require additional support; they also conclude that good practice and well-targeted interventions can have a positive impact (see for example Marsh and Cao 2005).

---

[11] This exercise is based on one featured in Fox and Arnull (2013: 61).

Nonetheless the studies indicate that while most parents who use drugs or alcohol to a harmful extent will try and care for their children, their ability to do so is impaired by regular or intensive drinking or drug use sessions, which affect both the ability to care and respond appropriately (EMCDDA 2010). As a result, numerous studies (ACMD 2003; Wales et al. 2009; UKDPC 2012; EMCDDA 2012b) have shown that children and young people whose parents are substance-dependent can appear withdrawn or preoccupied, appear to have few(er) friends or not engage with other young children effectively or may show a range or anxieties or worries beyond their years, thus:

- they may take on more responsibilities than one might normally expect (for example for household chores, shopping or care of siblings);

- they may also be anxious and worried, often concerned to get home because they worry about a parent when they are out or about getting home in case the parent is intoxicated and may have harmed themself or be unpleasant, difficult or violent;

- they may not want to take friends or others into their home because of parental unpredictability with regard to intoxication and feelings of shame about this and the stigma that may result;

- they may not want to take friends or others into the home because the home is in poor repair because money is spent on substances or the parent does not take pride in the home with concomitant feelings of shame or embarrassment;

- children experience more acute shame and embarrassment where the substance user is a mother or where use is illicit drugs rather than alcohol;

- children will go to considerable lengths to hide parental substance dependency and will see this as themselves managing or 'coping' with the situation: they strongly want to avoid the stigma associated with parental substance dependency;

- living with a substance-dependent parent is linked to some level of neglect, uncertainty and stress and in extreme cases violence and abuse;

- children raised by substance-dependent parents are more likely to develop substance use problems themselves.

Children may therefore display other factors that may be observed but poorly understood by a teacher or generic practitioner but are clearly indicative of a need for further investigation. In this vein a UK ChildLine report found that a child rarely phoned with the primary issue being the alcohol use of a parent, but that this often then emerged as an issue during the course of a call and where this occurred the alcohol use was seen as having a profound impact on their lives (Wales et al. 2009). Common to all generic practitioners therefore is the need to have good communication skills and in particular listening skills. If there are worries or concerns about a child, observe them, listen to them, give them time – allow them to tell you what is happening that makes them worried or anxious, ashamed or embarrassed.

Another important area where generic and treatment services need to be sensitive is the concern that those who have parental responsibility but are concerned about their own substance use feel about accessing treatment services. This may be because of childcare issues; for example it may mean that:

- they cannot access treatment services because they also have children with them;

- they cannot get an appointment during school time;

- they do not want their children/others in the family to know they consider their use problematic;

- they have serious (and legitimate concerns) that if they access treatment services there is the possibility that child protection issues will be raised and/or enquiries started.

The EMCDDA (2012a) report acknowledges that because of these factors, working with parents who use drugs or who are substance-dependent can be challenging. As a practitioner, therefore, it becomes even more important that you are able to be thoughtful and reflective, accurate and straightforward about any concerns or worries and accurate and straightforward about what is working well, where strengths are to be found and how those might be built on. You need to understand that the evidence is that treatment does have positive effects for many, but that the situation is complex. For example, Marsh and Cao (2005) found that the most predictive factor for reduced substance use 12 months after exiting treatment for parents was the frequency of the counselling (at least weekly) parents received during treatment; treatment duration of at least four months was important for all groups but only a significant predictor of positive outcomes for fathers (Marsh and Cao 2005: 1275). If a parent is accessing treatment you should therefore work with them to understand what type of service they are accessing, what they are being offered, whether it meets their needs, and whether there are other needs not being met. For example, Marsh and Cao (2005) suggest that while mothers were more likely to be offered 'ancillary' services such as housing advice than other types of service users, this was not frequently the case. Overall, therefore, the evidence indicates the need for a holistic assessment and treatment approach that looks at the range of factors contributing to the current situation that includes the substance dependency but is not so focused upon it that it is used to define the individual, family and their needs.

As a practitioner you need to be able to overcome hurdles, resistance or hostility that arise because of parental concerns about losing responsibility for their children[12] and/or children's worries that they have 'let their parents down' by not protecting them or because outside agencies have become involved because they voiced their concerns or fears. The EMCDDA (2012a) urges practitioners to engage in such a way that ensures that they seek to balance both the rights of the parent and the child. Clearly, within the UK the rights of the child are paramount (Children Act 2004), but it is nonetheless important as a practitioner to remain open-minded and consider that the child's needs may best be served by supporting parents who are experiencing difficulties, and noting that many children whose parents have substance use problems do not develop problems in later life (Velleman and Orford 1999). Thus, do not assume there is a problem or that the best option is to remove the child.[13]

---

[12] These sorts of issues are also encountered in practice with different groups; thus young care leavers who become parents report similar concerns about social work investigations (Arnull 2013b).

[13] See also, for example, guidance by Galvani and Forrester 2009 and www.swalcdrugs.com, a basic introductory website aimed at social workers in particular.

Despite all support, however, there are occasions when the needs of the child are best met by removing them from their parent or carer who is substance-dependent and this may not be in the interest of the adult, many of whom will then describe feeling as though they now have no reason to reduce or control their use and for whom the removal of the child signifies another 'failure'. These situations are extremely difficult and very sad, but they do occur in practice and the rights, needs and safety of the child do take precedence. In these situations, where possible, the adults should remain supported and able to access services so that they may come to see the removal as a step towards getting everything in place for them to be able to return to taking care of their children again when issues are resolved and the situation under their control, rather than a permanent step towards removal.

A pilot of specialist practice is the Family Drug and Alcohol Court (2011) in London, a specialist family court working with parents who are substance users and whose children are at risk of being taken into care. The evaluation report (Harwin et al. 2011) of effectiveness was a small study but its early indications were positive for the experimental group where:

*   more parents controlled their use than in the control group (48 per cent of mothers and 36 per cent of fathers);

*   parents were more likely to access treatment more quickly and more likely to stay in treatment and receive a broader range of services;

*   more parents were reunited with their children (39 per cent);

*   there were cost savings of £1,200 per family, fewer contested cases, and the researchers took the view that cases were conducted in a more constructive way – for example families liked the consistency of seeing the same judge.

In both the experimental and control group the average length of time it took for cases to progress through the court was the same; however, some children from the experimental group were reunited with their parents and in these instances the progress of the cases took longer. The positive early indications have therefore suggested that intensive support can help families to stay together and receive treatment and reduce substance use (Harwin et al. 2011).

The EMCDDA (2012) suggest that the same range of issues is relevant to pregnant substance users and the services that target them, for example arguing that:

> there is strong evidence that the provision of appropriate advice and support can improve the outcome for both mother and child.
>
> (EMCDDA 2012a: 16)

Pregnancy is also seen as an important opportunity for intervention as it is a point when families most need help; the EMCDDA (2012a) suggested that families were often open to assistance but the opportunity was missed because substance use or specialist services within maternity units were in general poorly developed. The EMCDDA (2012a) say that improving maternity services would be an important point for potential intervention because many studies highlight *the stress and social disruption that can result from having a family member with a drug problem* (EMCDDA 2012a: 16). Their conclusion is also that those working within this setting could do more to recognise signs of substance dependence and then support women and families to access specialist services and this is again resonant with other findings by Gilbert et al. (2009) and Leavey (2011) with regard to generic practice. In this setting the findings have particular resonance in the UK for those working as midwives and in antenatal and health visiting services.

The EMCDDA (2012a) posits that it will become increasingly important for prevention and harm reduction strategies to focus on the family because *a growing evidence base points to the effectiveness of broad-based prevention strategies that target both the environment and the individual* (EMCDDA 2012a: 14). They foresee such approaches as developing within a resiliency based framework suggesting that *stronger families may lower the risk of a range of problematic behaviours, including drug use* (EMCDDA 2012a: 14). It is this sort of area the family court seeks to address through a range of multi-agency and multi-professional interventions and support. The EMCDDA (2012a) are concerned, however, that:

> *Despite the positive findings for interventions in this area, the fact that they remain, to a large extent, poorly developed, highlights the more general problem that findings from research on prevention often fail to be translated into policies and practice.*
>
> (EMCDDA 2012a: 14)

The reasons for this are complex; services of this sort are not delivered by drug 'experts', but are delivered by a mix of professionals who may not understand how and where to lobby to demonstrate the effectiveness of their services at lowering or treating substance use problems or supporting substance users. Additionally, practitioners may not recognise that their practice is impacting upon substance use because that is not the area of practice upon which they place the most value and it may take many years for impacts from these holistic interventions to be shown and then it may be difficult to account for all variables. Finally, practitioners may not recognise the significance of the wider impacts, nor how to collect data or evidence them – the many evaluations of Sure Start encountered these sorts of difficulties until an RCT was able to show definitive improvements against specific areas (Eisenstadt 2013; Hutchings et al. 2007; Little 2007).

Nonetheless, given that the provision of support to pregnant women is almost universally provided in one form or another across Europe, interventions at this point do present a real opportunity for generic health and social care workers to be able to intervene to good effect. This means moreover that generic practitioners need to be aware enough of substance use issues to be able to 'spot' when they may be relevant as part of a generic assessment, be they a midwife, health visitor, generic social worker, obstetrician, etc. Furthermore the practitioner needs to know how to discuss the matter, how to refer appropriately and how to support the person/family – this means adopting an anti-oppressive, person-centred approach towards the service user (Fox and Arnull 2012; Thompson 2001). In so doing, practitioners can also ensure that within their organisations they support and ensure effective, equal, accessible and relevant support and services to all families/patients/service users.

Lastly, the findings from the EMCDDA (2012a) highlight the importance for generic practitioners across the health and social care spectrum to understand how in their practice, by establishing positive relationships with service users, they can support them to make broader and wider changes in their lives that may help them and others within their families to achieve more positive outcomes.

Older people

The older population both within the UK and across Europe and most parts of the world has traditionally had lower levels of drug use and drug trying. The reasons for this cover a whole range of complex and interwoven issues, but in part is related to lower levels of availability pre-war as well as lower levels of disposable income with which to socialise. However, social changes in the 1960s and the increasing use of a range of substances from that period onwards now mean that there are a growing number of older substance users, some of whom may or may not be dependent or have experienced dependency in the past, but find themselves with problems associated with their use as they age.

Prevalence figures for the older population are harder to come by as they are not always isolated from the overall totals and 'older' is a relative term; data from the USA suggest that just under 3 per cent of men and a smaller percentage of women have a 'diagnosable alcoholic condition' with about 20 per cent misusing alcohol and prescribed medication or showing signs of problematic use (Steinhagen and Freidman 2008). 'Older' is a relative term, but it is usually taken to mean those who are 50 or over. However, the EMCDDA (2012a) suggests within Europe that it may be helpful to consider those over 30 as 'older' substance users because of the health effects of prolonged and dependent use; in part because it is probable that they may also be presenting for treatment for the first time and to continue doing so for some time to come; moreover by the time they present to treatment they may be experiencing similar health effects to other 'older' drug users. Thus as the EMCDDA report (2012a) notes:

> *Opioid users entering specialist treatment are on average 33 years old, with female clients being younger in most countries. Across Europe, male opioid clients outnumber their female counterparts by a ratio of about three to one. The great majority of opioid clients report having started to use the drug before the age of 30, with almost half (46%) of all opioid clients having done so before the age of 20. In general, opioid users report higher levels of homelessness and unemployment and lower levels of education than primary users of other drugs, and they are usually concentrated in urban areas.*
>
> (EMCDDA 2012a: 72–3)

For those who are drug users and alcohol users and who have grown older and continued using it is probable that they will have accumulated a range of health and social effects. These may include liver and stomach/intestinal problems or liver failure for dependent alcohol users, some mental health problems such as depression, memory loss or psychosis and probable social isolation as the result of relationship problems and breakdown as the result of use. For dependent older drug users given past patterns of use and availability it is probable that they may have been an IV user and if this is the case they may have accumulated health issues along the way including a range of blood-borne infections such as hepatitis C and HIV/AIDS and/or problems with their veins, such as abscesses, resultant infections or collapsed veins, and a range of other health issues, such as a number of previous hospitalisation events related to overdose or poor quality drugs. Additionally, people who have been frequent or dependent users for a long time may find that the changes in their physiology as they age mean that their use, though unchanged, is now problematic to their health or social well-being. For those who continue to use intravenously the risk of drug-related death or infection remains.

Alongside those who have used substances all their lives are those who begin to use substances as they grow older. They may do this to counter health problems, such as pain, and find they are dependent on those thereafter; they make take sleeping tablets or anti-depressants because of difficulties sleeping which could be related to health or bereavement and again find they are dependent. They may drink alcohol because they enjoy it or to counter loneliness and again find they are increasingly dependent or experiencing other effects within their homes such as depression, confusion or falls, which can go undiagnosed or misdiagnosed because they are unwilling or ashamed to tell anyone and others do not suspect or ask about drug or alcohol use because the person is 'old' and they make the assumption that this would not be a factor nor problematic (EMCDDA 2012a; Steinhagen and Freidman 2008). Additionally people may not be drinking more but may find their bodies can no longer metabolise alcohol in the way they could previously and this becomes problematic, or they are now on prescribed medication with a contra or complicating effect. Equally, older people carry the same family histories as they did as young people and may also have family histories of substance use, depression and anxiety that they may become less resilient to withstand as they grow less physically or mentally able, become more isolated as the result of those effects or because people around them have died or moved away, or they have less access to financial and physical resources.

Steinhagen and Friedman (2008) note that the misuse of alcohol and prescribed medication are the most common forms of substance misuse and dependency in older people[14] for a number of reasons and say that the reasons this goes undiagnosed as frequently as it does is largely because of a lack of training and therefore recognition among medical and generic healthcare staff:

> *Even if providers are aware of the need to look for signs of substance abuse and misuse, they often lack the professional training or skills to recognize them in the older population. Signs and symptoms of alcohol abuse and misuse are similar to those of other common medical conditions and to what is often mistakenly believed to be part of the normal aging process. They include memory problems, fatigue, sleep problems, confusion, depression, anxiety, and irritability. Signs of medication misuse include mood changes, irritability, lack of energy and concentration, loss of short-term memory, and general loss of interest.*
>
> *In addition, many retired elders drink unnoticed at home or in local bars or social settings. They are not nearly as likely to get in trouble with the law or their places of employment as younger people. Many older adults and their family members don't realize that they have a drinking problem or are misusing medications. And when they do, they often feel shame or guilt and don't want to be stigmatized as alcoholics or drug addicts are. Family members may also fail to view drinking*

---

[14] Recent figures in 2013 for admissions to hospital for 'poisoning' suggest a similar pattern for women where levels of admission as the result of poisoning arising from prescribed medication far exceeded those for illicit substances: www.thesundaytimes.co.uk/sto/news/uk_news/Health/article1304729.ece

or medication abuse as harmful. For all these reasons, many older adults with sub-stance use problems don't seek the help they need.

As a result of failures of screening, lack of training in the signs and symptoms of sub-stance misuse, stigma, ageist assumptions, and ignorance about substance abuse problems among older adults, such problems often go undiagnosed and untreated.

They suggest that assessment and intervention therefore requires a different approach:

engaging older adults in substance abuse treatment, it's important to understand that older adults who do not have a history of lifelong, hard-core addiction are usu-ally reluctant to be associated with what are stereotypically known as down-and-out alcoholics or drug addicts. They need to be understood and treated in contexts that are more comfortable for them.

Their findings and recommendations have resonance for those in the UK working in district nursing for example. What will therefore stand you in good stead as a generic practitioner is an open mind, a willingness to consider all options, an ability to use your communica-tion skills to discuss and assess the issues at hand and an anti-oppressive, person-centred approach which allows you to think with the service user what interventions might be called for and how best that support can be accessed.

Prisoners

There are continuing concerns across Europe that despite significant changes introduced over the recent past to target drug use and its links with crime, a high number of those who use substances, and especially those who use them problematically, will end up in prison; this is especially true of those who are poor and also dependent drug or alcohol users. Many offenders have experienced multiple problems and victimisations and will have a complex history that will then form part of their treatment needs (Fox and Arnull 2013; UKDPC 2012); those needs will potentially be composed of health, welfare, substance use and criminogenic factors that may need to be addressed separately or together (UKDPC 2012; Arnull and Eagle 2009; Arnull et al. 2007).

A Home Affairs Committee report (2012) notes that:

* 70 per cent of offenders report drug misuse prior to prison;

* 51 per cent report drug dependency;

* 35 per cent admit injecting behaviour;

* 36 per cent report heavy drinking;

* 16 per cent are alcohol dependant.

The NTA (2012) similarly noted that there were approximately 130,000 people admitted to prison every year in England and Wales of whom about 70 per cent were drug users; they noted that a busy remand wing might see about 3,000 dependent drug users each year. It can be seen therefore that drug use among those who find themselves in prison is more common than for the general population and more likely to be linked to possible harms, for example injecting and heavy drinking, etc. The Home Affairs Committee also draws upon the findings of the Prison Reform Trust (2012) which found that 19 per cent of prisoners had used heroin for the *first* time in prison.

There are improvements, for example those found testing positive for drugs in prison has now fallen to 7.1 per cent (2010–11) from a high of over 24 per cent (1996–7). This appears to be the result of improved services in prison and the criminal justice system, which as we saw emerged post-TDTBB (1998) as a result of concerns about links between offending and substance use; thus, many treatment services were developed that were available within the CJS or accessed via them. The Home Affairs Committee report (2012) notes significant improvements:

- Funding for prison drug treatment was in 2010 over 15 times greater than in 1997 – with record numbers engaging in treatment.

- During the same period, drug use in prisons, as measured by random mandatory drug tests, decreased by 68 per cent.

- This was accompanied by a significant decline in adult reoffending since 2000, with a fall of 13 per cent between 2005 and 2006.

- Since the establishment of the Drug Intervention Programme (DIP) in 2002, to provide a route out of crime and into treatment, recorded acquisitive crime – of which drug-related crime constitutes a large proportion – has fallen by almost a third.

The UKDPC in a 2008 review and then reiterated in their final report (2012: 126–8) high-lighted that there was a need for two things – diversion and community punishments – rather than the use of imprisonment for 'drug-dependent offenders' and the improvement of prison drug services, which should be linked into community services. The latter included their wel-coming the rolling out of the Integrated Drug Treatment System (IDTS) and the use of Drug Recovery Wings in prisons, which was also voiced by the Home Affairs Committee report (2012). UKDPC (2012) also recommended better identification and assessment systems for people entering prison, ensuring healthcare meets national standards set by the National Institute for Health and Care Excellence (NICE), enhancing the performance management of prison treatment services and ensuring continuity of care between prison and the commu-nity. The relevance of the latter is always highlighted, both because people may begin good work in prisons that is interrupted by their release and they may be returning to an area or community in which they have not lived substance-free or interacted with treatment ser-vices for some time; additionally, release from prison is a time where there is significant and enhanced risk of relapse into use and overdose and death.

The NTA (2012) laid out what was expected in terms of identification, assessment and treat-ment when a drug user was imprisoned:

- *The substance misuse team arranges treatment for any prisoner with a drug or alcohol problem. This includes psychosocial therapies (to encourage positive behaviour change) and/or medication (like detoxification, or substitute prescribing for opiate addicts). Detoxification is the most common prescribing response in local prisons.*

- *Prisoners should receive regular reviews to check progress on their treatment goals and ensure links with appropriate community treatment and support services upon release.*

- *Most drug-dependent prisoners are on short-term sentences (less than six months) that are not long enough to effectively tackle dependence. However, those on longer sentences are expected to get off drugs and work towards recovery while in custody.*

- *Prisoners dependent on heroin are typically prescribed opiate substitute medicines such as methadone or buprenorphine. Revised clinical guidelines in April 2010 limited open-ended prescribing of substitute medication in prisons.*

- *Close working between prison and community services ensures continuity of care, and reduces the costly revolving door of relapse, reoffending and re-imprisonment.*

Many dependent substance users who are in prison will have a number of health and mental health issues some or all of which will be related to their substance use. Quite often this is because by the time substance use has become so problematic that it involves offending or behaviour problematic to others the person has been using long enough, and often without support or treatment, to have developed the sorts of health and psychosocial affects we discussed earlier. Despite a well-tracked and highly developed evidence base concerning dependent substance users and prisons the EMCDDA also reports that:

> *Rarely do prisons offer a standard of care equivalent and comparable to that provided to the wider community.*
>
> (EMCDDA 2012a: 17)

There have been recent reviews of drug treatment within the CJS such as Lord Bradley's review on diversion (2009) and Lord Patel's report on prison drug treatment (2010). The Centre for Mental Health, DrugScope and UKDPC (2012) in a joint report noted that there was the possibility for the *role of 'offender health' within the emerging commissioning landscape* to include *opportunities for 'joined up' approaches and for the identification of dual diagnosis as a strategic priority*. However, current legislation in the UK introduced in the Health and Social Care Act (2012) required from April 2013 substance use treatment services to be provided to the same standards and levels of treatment or to be equitable with those to be found in the community; the NHS Commissioning Board (NCB) is now responsible for drug and alcohol treatment in prison and LAs are responsible for treatment in the community using a ring-fenced public health grant from PHE (Strang 2012). As a result there have been real concerns voiced by the NTA (2012) and others that in fact this splitting of the treatment system would lead to difficulties and a loss of the very real gains made under the IDTS. Clearly the recent nature of these changes means this is a developing process and one which may well be affected by privatisation, PbR and budget cuts.

Mental health and 'dual diagnosis'

As we have seen in our discussion of young people, cannabis use and psychosis, mental health difficulties and substance misuse are two conditions that can coexist, interrelate, exacerbate, hide or disguise one another. The coexistence of mental health issues and substance misuse, dependency or difficulties is often referred to as 'dual diagnosis'.

In a discussion document reflecting on changing government policies affecting drug users with mental health problems and thus those most frequently referred to as having a 'dual diagnosis', the Centre for Mental Health, DrugScope and UKDPC (2012) noted that other recent research such as the Co-morbidity of Substance Misuse and Mental Illness Collaborative study or COSMIC1 (2002) had shown that:

- *75 per cent of users of drug services and 85 per cent of users of alcohol services were experiencing mental health problems;*

- *30 per cent of the drug treatment population and over 50 per cent of those in treatment for alcohol problems had 'multiple morbidity';*

- *38 per cent of drug users with a psychiatric disorder were receiving no treatment for their mental health problem;*

- *44 per cent of mental health service users either reported drug use or were assessed to have used alcohol at hazardous or harmful levels in the past year.*

They also drew attention to another study undertaken in 2002 by Strathdee, which had found that:

- *dual diagnosis was present in 20 per cent of community mental health clients; 43 per cent of psychiatric in-patients; 56 per cent of people in secure services;*

- *the group identified as dually diagnosed had worse physical health, higher levels of personality disorder, greater levels of disability, greater risk profiles and lower quality of life than those who were not identified as having a dual diagnosis.*

They also drew on the Prison Reform Trust (2010), which had reported that 75 per cent of all prisoners had a dual diagnosis.

The scale and nature of the issue of intertwined mental health and substance use issues and difficulties are therefore substantial across both populations and as we have seen in the discussions of confounded factors for cannabis use and psychosis and for substance misuse and the elderly, the difficulty can be understanding what came first: the mental health difficulty or the substance use. However, as a generic practitioner it is not really required that you solve this conundrum with a service user; what is important is a recognition that there may be a number of competing or coexisting factors that need to be considered when undertaking assessments, considering referrals and thinking about potential sources of intervention. There is now clear guidance that

> *mental health services were responsible for ensuring anyone with a severe mental health problem and a substance misuse problem were their responsibility and that integrated care was the norm for this group.*

> (DoH 2002)

There are also other guidance documents such as *A Guide for the Management of Dual Diagnosis in Prisons* (DoH and Ministry of Justice 2009).

Experts in the area are in general keen to have the complexity of the issues understood and have some concerns about current directions of travel, such as the different forms of commissioning for prisons and community drug interventions as the result of the Health and Social Care Act (2012). Reflecting on current issues and particular PbR schemes the Centre for Mental Health, DrugScope and UKDPC (2012) said:

our understanding is that people with 'dual diagnosis' are explicitly excluded from the drug and alcohol recovery PBR pilots. If the two payment systems being developed do not combine fully or leave out significant groups of people, they will create barriers to better services rather than encouraging improved care for all.

There are therefore real concerns, especially as the dual diagnosis population is often also intertwined with the offending population, which adds a further layer of complexity and potentially also stigmatisation and isolation.

As a generic practitioner the guidance once again is to be open-minded and reflective in your assessment; work with the service user to understand and develop an accurate picture of the range of issues and difficulties they face and the strengths that they have; use this to think with them about the next steps and where best they may be referred or assisted. It is probable that if your initial assessment is correct mental health services may have direct responsibility, but recognise that service users can be resistant to such suggestions in the first instance because of the stigmatisation they may feel such a referral might bring. Work in this area is extremely likely to involve significant multi-agency liaison and partnership working and this will also include working with the service user in a partnership-based approach; this is considered to be the most effective method for intervention and underpins all of the good practice guidance in this area.

6 Approaches to substance use

Introduction

This chapter presents the dominant treatment and intervention approaches to substance misuse. It discusses the theories and the underpinning values to help the reader 'find' themselves and where relevant their practice within this context. The discussion focuses on harm reduction and dependency concepts and addiction concepts. It introduces the reader to the way these influence and underpin the various forms of intervention on offer: for example motivational interviewing (MI) and 12-step programmes.

The chapter will also describe the elements or 'layers' of treatment that until very recently have been called 'tiers' for treatment and commissioning (Strang 2012). What 'layers' and 'tiers' attempt to describe is the type and range of interventions that can be found, the sorts of practitioners who would be involved at each stage and the type and depth of knowledge they would need. In order to help the reader to visualise and conceptualise how this applies to practice they will also be presented in table form. Again, where relevant the generic practitioner can then also use this as a basis from which to develop their practice using the table as a basic tool for consideration of whether they have the skills, resources and knowledge to support the service user or whether they need to consider referring someone for more specialist support. It can also be used as a tool with service users to think through with them the issues arising and the support required. This therefore provides a basic assessment tool that can be used to support assessment strategies.

LEARNING OUTCOMES

In this chapter we will therefore cover:

» The dominant treatment approaches.

» Theories and underpinning values.

»   *Types of treatment and the range of practitioners involved.*

»   *A basic, initial assessment toolkit.*

By the end of this chapter you should be able to:

»   *Describe the dominant treatment approaches to drug and alcohol use in the UK.*

»   *Critically evaluate the key theoretical approaches.*

»   *Critically analyse how theoretical debates influence practice approaches.*

»   *Demonstrate your critical understanding and reflection on assessment in order to provide support for those who use drug and alcohol services.*

The dominant treatment approaches

The dominant treatment approaches are informed either by a social model or by a medical model. In reality the two are not as distinct as this would suggest and while there are practitioners who ascribe to only one approach, many actually see the value and criticality that both bring. This is especially so because it is unclear what causes substance dependency or, in fact, enables or supports people who are drug or alcohol-dependent to give up (Keys et al. 2006; UKDPC 2012).

Practitioners should also be open to the fact that service users and those who are drug or alcohol-dependent may take a different view about what will aid their recovery from that they take; unless a person is working in a very distinct, ideological setting this is usually the case. Thus as a probation officer I supported many drug users into 12-step rehabilitative programmes and helped them to locate and access Alcoholics Anonymous (AA) and Narcotics Anonymous (NA), whose approaches are also informed by 12 steps and include views of a 'higher power' and a belief that 'once an alcoholic always an alcoholic'; although my own perspective was quite different, I saw many people for whom this approach was useful.

Both AA and NA are powerful, service-user led treatment approaches and my notions of open, person-focused practice which sought to be anti-oppressive and inclusive and which aimed to support and facilitate the person to be able to make their own choice of how to seek to deal with the problems they were experiencing, the dependence on the substance which they felt and the desire to tackle and change this meant I did not consider it was for me to discount choices they made; I considered my role was to respect the choices the service user made about the best way to be supported. What underpinned my practice therefore was a belief in the right of the service user to self-determination, which is in line with social work values (BASW 2012: 2.2;[1] IFSW 2012: 4.1.1). I also took the view that what was important was that someone was able to find what worked for them and

[1] http://cdn.basw.co.uk/upload/basw_112315-7.pdf and http://ifsw.org/policies/statement-of-ethical-principles/accessed 23 July 2013.

that whatever worked and assisted was valuable. The fact that I found evidence that suggested that structural, environmental and cultural factors were greater contributory factors to drug trying and taking than anything else, did not mean that I felt I should, could or would impose my analytical perspective on others. I did share my views with service users and talked in detail with them about the different approaches to problematic, dependent use and terms like 'addiction' with the intention of assisting them to think about what would feel comfortable, supportive and 'right' for them. In my experience people always found this approach helpful; it is something they will have pondered on when considering whether they needed help, how they might access it and what it might mean – clear, non-judgemental information allowed them to think about what they might choose, were they to choose.

The social model

The social model is most likely to be associated with the concepts and language of dependence, rather than addiction. It is derived from sociological and ethnographic theory, from social policy and criminology and some parts of psychology; in addition some health and medical practitioners will also take this view (Galvani 2012; UKDPC 2012; Goodman 2007; Bourgois et al. 2006).

It is probable that many academics, policy-makers and practitioners coming from this perspective will see structural factors, such as poverty, employment and educational opportunities, housing, social, environmental and structural supports (such as benefits, access to health and treatment) as important in influencing the likelihood of drug and alcohol use, the likelihood of that use being problematic, and influencing the opportunities for recovery. Social models of substance use, misuse and dependence may include seeing the behaviours as:

- socially learned and thus able to be 'unlearned';

- legitimate, exploratory and risk-taking behaviour common to human experience and similar to people choosing to do rock climbing, drive too fast, sail single-handedly around the world or ride horses, all of which include some unnecessary level of risk-taking, and a search for a 'thrill', an unusual experience and a pushing of boundaries of human experience;

- a legitimate and logical response to structural, social, psychological or other oppression, experience or abuse.

Academics, researchers, policy-makers and practitioners whose views support this theory base, do not discount that some biological, neurophysiological or other factors may play a role. However, they are usually inclined to interpret the evidence as showing that there is no evidence to suggest that these factors are in any way definitive or explanatory, although they may be contributory.

The social model is most likely to see drug and alcohol use and dependence as broader than the individual themselves – it looks at contextual, structural and social factors, as well as biological and physiological ones (Bourgois 2003, 2008). For many proponents and supporters of this perspective this is the key factor that influences their analysis.

Some have argued that the social model, like the medical model, can be limiting, merely concerned with factors that influence the likelihood of drug use/dependence, rather than concerned with those factors that might *constitute and underpin* it (Keys et al. 2006: 66), but this critique seems at odds with the broader analytical perspective taken.

The social model is a common social policy, research and academic approach (UKDPC 2012: 109); it is most likely to be influenced and derived from post-positivist or qualitative research theory and methods. Those interested in the social model may well be interested in how social factors, economic problems and structural constraints lead to or contribute to problematic drug or alcohol use, influence and affect the choices people can make or consider are available to them and thus understand why problematic use may be more common in certain parts of the population – they are inclined to interpret this evidence as causally related to those social factors. Research influenced by this perspective is therefore most likely to prioritise or include interviews with substance users and may look at how people moved into use, how they became dependent and how they move away from use or their reasons for using/choosing not to use. Nonetheless, much of the research that has been influential in the UK and beyond the 1990s, eg by Pearson (1991), Bourgois (2003, 2008), Bourgois and Schonberg (2007), Parker et al. (1998) and Dunlap (1995) on structural and economic factors, and Home Office (2002), Bennett (2001), Edmunds et al. (1998), NTORS (Department of Health 1996), Gossop et al. (2001) and Hough et al. (1995) regarding links between drugs and crime, will also have come from this perspective and much of that includes at least some quantitative research methods; thus it will be composed of post-positivist elements.

Understanding this is important when reading research on substance use: it is not easy to form a simple judgement on the nature of the research. For example, research that I and a team undertook for the NTA on crack users of drug treatment services used quantitative and qualitative elements; the methodology for the quantitative elements was devised by an expert in using quantitative approaches and allowed us to consider the possible impacts of the social intervention programmes (Arnull et al. 2007). This was a developing area, however, and some did not understand or misunderstood the approach and/or the findings. Quantitative and mixed methods approaches are now better understood and although methodological debates and arguments continue many have accepted (especially those commentating from a medical background) what experts in the area of quantitative methods and the social arena told them at the time, that designing a perfect RCT in this area would be extremely difficult and other methods might be more or at least as helpful (Bourgois et al. 2006).

RCT methods are useful for considering whether an *input* (ie a substitute drug) had an *outcome or effect* (ie did all of those who took the substitute drug cease to use drugs while all of those in the control group continued to use?). The difficulty, as the reader will appreciate, is that with the complexity of factors implicated in substance use and a person's life it is hard to be sure that just one *input* was responsible for the *outcome*, unless of course the findings were as extreme as I suggest when you might look very hard at all other variables and consider this was the case![2] Thus although both the HO and DoH during the late 1990s

---

[2] This is an extremely simplified description of an RCT method; it is a positivist research method, frequently used in medical trials. Some such as the Cochrane group have upheld it as a 'gold standard'

adopted research scales that privileged RCT and quantitative methods, in fact much mixed method and qualitative work has continued, been funded and found useful. This appears to be in part due to the difficulties that have been experienced in attempting RCTs in the social world and in part due to a better and more sophisticated understanding of how to use research and think about what might work, for some people in some circumstances[3] (Bourgois et al. 2006). Paylor et al. (2012: 20) draw out the difficulty in a brief discussion on what implications the debate about the most efficacious research methods has for evidence-based policy-making. The trend across all academic disciplines to be more cautious about what they 'know', sits more comfortably with post-positivist and critical assumptions about the world, but is also echoed by 'hard' physical scientists such as Professor Athene Donald, whose scientific work seeks to work harder to understand complexity and thus *understanding structure-function-processing relationships*[4] – essentially this is what much research on substance use seeks to do, whether coming from a social or a medical model as we shall discuss below.

In terms of practice the social model is used and has been influential in establishing the foundation of, for example, harm minimisation models, premised on notions of self-determination and a non-judgemental approach to intervention. It is also usually entwined with a conception of personal agency,[5] which assumes that the individual, to some extent, regardless of social, cultural and environmental factors, has the ability to choose or decide. Thus an individual can choose whether or not to use drugs and alcohol on the basis of whatever knowledge and information they have; and if they use them to consider whether or not their use has become dependent or problematic and where that is the case to choose to seek help and support to stop and put dependence behind them, or ameliorate the problematic effects and minimise harms.

The social model is therefore most likely to emphasise the ability of the person/substance user to change their own behaviour through their own agency, along with appropriate support they can choose. Thus, for example, in the coverage of drug consumption rooms some argue that simply by being there and offering a supportive service alternative options are modelled, which people are then at liberty to take up, without the notion being thrust on them (*The Observer*, 5 May 2013).

research method and it was linked to evidence-based medicine and to a lesser extent evidence-based practice. This contention is considered by many to be reductionist, is hotly and increasingly contested and disputed and the evidence suggests its ineffectiveness as an approach in some areas and the effectiveness of other research approaches in some areas.

[3] For example, the Youth Justice Board's Effective Practice Classification Panel established in 2012 to consider research and provide guidance for practitioners about how likely it may be useful to them is established on the basis of a broad understanding of research and its usefulness.

[4] www.bss.phy.cam.ac.uk/~amd3

[5] Agency is a concept derived from philosophy and subsequently used in sociology and humanistic psychology. Generic practitioners will usually have come across the term previously as it is a common theoretical proposition in the underpinning social sciences to much health and social care work. Agency as a concept implies the ability of an individual to 'act' in a way they determine. In itself it implies no moral action/condition/factor. Some regard agency as being affected by different factors, eg structural = Marx and structural or sociological explanations; the subconscious = Freud and the psychodynamic school; predetermined or stimuli response = behaviourist school; inner feelings and self-concept = humanists and the humanist psychology of Carl Rogers and Abraham Maslow.

The picture has currently been further complicated by policy reviews such as the most recent led by Strang (2012) regarding treatment approaches for opioid users in the UK; the review promulgates the adoption of a 'recovery' model. This model is essentially holistic and refers to 'layers' of treatment responses that tackle different areas of someone's life and which may all be relevant to their substance use. The review and its recommendations will form the basis for future commissioning of treatment services aimed at opioid users, but appears anecdotally to be affecting the review of all treatment systems and their commission – in this respect therefore it becomes relevant in local areas.

However, this review, undertaken for the outgoing NTA, was peopled almost entirely by those from a medical perspective and the term 'addiction' is freely used. This represents a change to policy document language in the UK and the backgrounds of those playing a principal role in drug policy, suggesting a resurgence of health-led approaches. Surprisingly therefore, the model proposed is one that is holistic and referred to by practitioners as a 'social' model – as ever, therefore, the substance use policy and practice world remains complex and often confusing.

The medical model

The medical model is derived from Western, developed countries' conceptions of medicine and health and has been influenced by that theoretical base. It usually considers that dependent substance use is a 'disease' and it will use this conceptualisation to talk about dependence and problematic use and recovery.

Research in this area is most likely to be derived from positivist conceptions of knowledge and much research from this perspective will be influenced by this approach – eg RCTs, drug trials, brain scanning and imaging, etc. However, 12-step and other programmes have drawn extensively on the testament of ex-users that this approach worked for them and are therefore more qualitative in their understanding of process and change (see, for example, high profile exponents like the British comedian Russell Brand (2013[6]) who also freely uses terms like 'addiction' and 'addict'). Therefore, as discussed above, use caution when reading research and do not assume that the methodological approach taken necessarily indicates the underpinning philosophical perspective.

The medical model is usually associated with notions of 'addiction' and most often presents problematic or repeated drug use as a physiological dependence. Drugs that do not create physiological dependency, such as cocaine, were a challenge to this view as some users considered themselves dependent – this was a key element initially in treatment services not engaging with cocaine and crack users and formed the background to the research I and others undertook (Arnull et al. 2007). Since that time notions of addiction have been adapted and grown to include psychological as well as physiological dependence. Addiction is usually seen as outside of the person's control, because they are 'diseased' and thus 'addicted'; its proponents are also more likely to be interested in and to investigate biological conceptions and explanations for drug and alcohol-dependent use.

[6] www.bbc.co.uk/programmes/p00wq21g: BBC 3 TV Programme 'Russell Brand: from addiction to recovery'. There are numerous other links to Russell Brand talking about his own substance use for 2013 including an appearance on BBC's Question Time.

'Addiction' is a term that has been used throughout history and there is evidence of its use in the Middle Ages (Withington 2013; Berridge 2007). It has dropped in and out of fashion over time, but currently is a fashionable term used to provide an explanation for a considerable range of behaviours; those are frequently based around the experience of sensation or sensation seeking. Those who use the term addiction consider the user/sensation seeker cannot stop/has no control over their behaviour and thus requires treatment and professional intervention (although see discussion about AA and NA). Addiction is therefore a term that has also been used to account for sexual behaviour, eating and violent sexual behaviour and has been offered as an explanatory factor for the behaviour of celebrities such as Tiger Woods (golfer), Russell Brand (comedian and actor), Paul Gascoigne (footballer) and Amy Winehouse (singer and song-writer).

As an explanatory term addiction suggests that the individual has no agency, no control and therefore cannot change; an individual may be enabled to change by a 'higher power', which may be a god or a practitioner or other service users or 'ex-addicts'. What we know, however, is that it is not true. An individual can achieve control and change by themselves and many cease to use substances and do so under their own power at some point (UKDPC 2012); in response to this evidence addiction has become modified as a term over time. Some medical proponents of addiction do seek to explain addictive, compulsive behaviour in terms of physical and psychological reactions; however, few seek to describe this as wholly explanatory in itself.

Research looking at the attributions substance users and non-substance users give for their own and others' behaviours supported previous findings, that terms like 'addict' are often self-ascribed by substance users where they consider their own use to be problematic (Monk and Heim 2011). These authors argue that the label is for the substance user 'functional' – in that it can both ascribe or remove guilt (2011: 649); labelling oneself an 'addict' could seem counterproductive implying that *one's free will is to a greater or lesser degree impaired*, but it might also remove personal responsibility with *blame diminished, thus protecting one's self-esteem* (Monk and Heim 2011: 645). The findings and their congruence with others regarding self-image and substance use are relevant to generic practitioners who should be aware of and think through the possible consequences that help-seeking might have. If you are supporting or 'nudging' someone to consider help in seeking treatment it is probable that they may also begin to call into question many notions they have formed about themselves and their own behaviour, many justifications and explanations. Change, treatment and help may challenge some of their notions that they are not responsible for the way things are or that they did not make choices that have contributed to where they are. Be sensitive to that, think through how best you can support them to adapt to those possibilities and make changes – in my experience this was especially painful for parents where they had lost the care of their children or more generally with regard to family/important other relationships.

Theory and underpinning values: social and medical explanations

The picture is very mixed about the influence of biological, physiological, psychological, social, cultural, economic and structural factors. These mechanisms are currently imperfectly understood and for some people in some circumstances different factors appear to offer an explanation; however, for others they do not. Like other areas of scientific investigation at this time we can 'see' the physiological effects of substances on the brain through scans and images, but although we can witness mechanisms and effects we do not currently have the knowledge to explain them.[7]

There is no doubt that while we can see the effects of certain substances on people's brain patterns these offer little or no explanation for their social behaviour. Alcohol use is widespread. Most people drink alcohol with no ill effect, socially, medically or otherwise, but for some there are ill effects and for others these are significant and profound – socially, mentally and biologically – the substance in itself does not offer the answer. For some, serious structural disadvantage, exclusion and oppression are clearly contributory factors to the choices they make and feel able to make and that may make substance use and/or dependency appear an attractive, possible or probable choice – others never experience that. Bourgois et al. (2006) and Bourgois (2003, 2008) explore how explanations for use/ addiction are mediated by ethnicity, poverty and other structural factors in their study of the practice of substance use in the USA. The picture is therefore complex – the important thing for the reader is to reflect upon it and to be open to explanations whatever your basic, explanatory preference.

Theory to practice: evidence, effectiveness and managing change

Much has changed with regard to substance use treatment in the last 25 years, post-TDT (1995), both within the UK and outside of it. For about ten years drug use and drug trying appeared to increase, but since then they have fallen fairly steadily and consistently as we have seen in previous chapters. There has also been a significant increase in the range and number of drug users coming into the drug treatment system and increasing evidence that there appears to be a 'treatment effect', thus that seeking help and accessing treatment seems to reduce substance use (see, for example, Marsden et al. 2009).

Prior to 1995, drug treatment followed a model of statutory and non-statutory delivery with medical models being more common in the former and social models in the latter. Drug treatment services were poorly funded and largely treated white male opiate users. With a changing pattern of drug use and users this was no longer acceptable and in addition it was challenged on the basis of oppressive and discriminatory practice. A study undertaken for the NTA on crack use and users, the availability and accessibility of treatment and the development and trialling of a new and specific model of treatment was funded as part of the activities incorporated in the Crack Action Plan (2002). The NTA recruited sites to the Crack Treatment Delivery Model (CTDM) pilot by inviting drug treatment services around the country to participate and the research was undertaken by the Policy & Practice Research Group (PPRG) based at Middlesex University. The NTA had emphasised to services that the pilot offered an opportunity to provide services based on *contemporary best practice and the available evidence base*, along with *having the opportunity to make existing opiate-based services relevant to the needs of a more diverse client group*; it also offered an opportunity

---

[7] This is true of other areas of scientific investigation, see for example work by Athene Donald, a Professor of Physics at Cambridge.

to meet with *other services to explore options for development*. The agencies chosen were mostly drawn from a list of *high crack areas* (Arnull et al. 2007: 9, 10) and the pilot included 13 drug services in 11 cities in the UK. It found that:

* The appropriateness of the service was important to service users (particularly women and those from BME groups) and affected their decision to attend for treatment.

* Service users placed a priority on fast access to treatment.

* All 13 services adapted some or all of the resource materials to local needs.

* Staff who adopted and adapted the materials were most positive about the pilot and most likely to consider they would continue using the new working practices and materials.

The pilot was adopted very differently across all 13 Tier 2 and 3 services,[8] in part because the treatment services themselves varied so much and in part because those engaging in the pilot had not been required to adopt the programme in just one form, ie there was no required programme/model integrity. This meant it was difficult to quantify impact in treatment outcomes and attribute them solely to the CTDM. Nonetheless, there were noticeable changes in the drug-using behaviour, health and offending between the first and second round of interviews for those 68 users across all sites who were interviewed twice.

* There was a statistically significant reduction in crack (and heroin) use for habitual users.

* There was an improvement across all five health groupings for males and across four groupings for females.

* Levels of offending were reduced.

* There were small improvements across all treatment domains.

The implications were:

* that there may have been a treatment effect;

* that appropriate treatment could help to reduce high levels of crack use;

* that there were quantifiable health benefits for those in treatment. (Arnull et al. 2007: 7, 8)

It is perhaps hard to appreciate now, that there was any debate about providing treatment to crack users or the gains for them by so doing. Furthermore, as respondents to another study by Arnull in 2007 testified, drug treatment had been aimed at the 'nice' users ie those who would submit to tests, long waiting times and imposed conditions – they were commonly white, male and opioid users. Those who were otherwise deemed unacceptable were offenders, for example, or those using the 'wrong' type of substance, for example crack or cocaine users found themselves unable to access services. Because treatment services were mainly aimed at white men in their 20s and 30s, it was difficult for women, BME groups and young people to access treatment and it was often posited

---

[8] Tiers of services are explained later in the chapter.

therefore that they did not experience drug problems requiring treatment or that for some reason specific to that group they were unsuitable or unwilling to access or engage in treatment. As Hayes (NTA 2013) comments, the drug strategies, and pilots like CTDM and many other activities, effectively tackled this state of affairs. But the situation in 2001 was as follows:

> The dominant political issue was waiting times. The average wait of nine weeks masked waits of many months across the country for particular types of treatment. Lengthy waits dissuaded many users from even trying to get into treatment, and sapped the motivation of those who did, resulting in high rates of non-attendance when people eventually reached the front of the queue.

> The service offered to the minority who made it into the system was patchy. Poor prescribing practice, unresponsive staff and inflexible working practices resulted in half of those who accessed treatment dropping out within the first few weeks.

> In many services standardised methadone withdrawal programmes were still commonplace and a significant proportion of individuals had their treatment terminated for failing to comply with the regime.

> Only a trickle of individuals successfully completed treatment.

Hayes (NTA 2013) highlights what underpinned the scale of change in treatment services:

> The challenge to the nascent NTA at its first Board meeting was to deploy the extra resources the government had pledged to channel into treatment – from £50m a year to £360m a year over the Parliament, in a way which addressed the deficits in the current system to deliver positive outcomes.

As the outgoing CEO of the NTA in 2013 he noted these gains since 2001:

> Today we can judge the impact of that investment and the extent to which the promise of the evidence has been achieved. Drug treatment services are much more efficient, effective and tailored to the needs of service users than they were in 2001. Local systems are better joined up, offering options for service users with a wider range of drug dependency problems and increasingly integrating health, criminal justice and wider support services. Access to mutual aid has improved significantly, prison based treatment is now expected to be delivered to the same standards as that in the community. Young people's interventions are available across the country and integrated into the broad range of services young people need.

> Average waits are now counted in days rather than months, the proportion of drug misusers who can access treatment is one of the highest in the world. Premature punitive discharge is no longer accepted practice and the proportion of those in treatment who drop out early is less than a third of what it was in 2001.

> The impact on outcomes is no less dramatic. A 2009 study in The Lancet demonstrated the significant reduction in opiate and crack use that occurs on treatment commencement and is subsequently sustained while individuals are retained.

The findings from *The Lancet* study show the same trends as for the CTDM; that contact with treatment services appears to reduce the health-related harms linked to substance use. The treatment services available for substance users have changed rapidly between 2001 and

2013, propelled by a huge increase in budget, focus and collection of data and evidence about what works, for whom and in what circumstances – it can be difficult to recall these are recent and important gains.

EXERCISE

Undertake a review of the substance use treatment services available in your area of practice, or the area in which you live, the services available within them and the drug users they seek to treat or refer. Add two additional columns to the table you have: the first for reflection and another for noting when the service, range of treatment options within it or a broader range of service users started. It is highly probable that in the very recent past the range of service provision and accessibility you can evidence now simply would not have been available.

Types of treatment

Tiers of treatment referred to the harm and level of need they were supposed to meet; thus Tier 1 services were those aimed at information gathering and often staffed by generic, or non-specialist staff; alternatively Tier 4 services were specialist services, usually in-patient and delivered by practitioners who specialised in substance use across a range of professional groups.

Tiers of treatment were introduced in Models of Care by the NTA in 2002 to make more intelligible the steps and ways through treatment and to enable commissioners of services to specify the level and type of service they were contracting. Most drug services are commissioned locally by the DAT, although complex services required at a national level (previously Tier 4) were often commissioned as part of a wider public health purchasing commitment. In 2006 the NTA updated the Models of Care guidance in part because:

> In Models of Care 2002, the four tiers were based upon a combination of setting, interventions and the agency responsible for providing the interventions. This has led to some differing interpretations and particularly over-rigid interpretation. In Models of Care: Update 2006, the tiers describe drug 'interventions' and the context for those interventions is described.

In 2010 in response to the new Drug Strategy (2010) and a fashion for 'recovery' models the NTA commissioned a new review of treatment for opioid/heroin users. What the *Medications in Recovery* (Strang 2012) document has to say essentially about the 'recovery' model is that while entering treatment, reducing substance use and dependence on substitute prescriptions are good things and evidence of 'progress in recovery' they are not evidence of 'recovery' itself; this it is argued is constituted thus:

> Recovery is a broader and more complex journey that incorporates overcoming dependence, reducing risk-taking behaviour and offending, improving health, functioning as a productive member of society and becoming personally fulfilled. These recovery outcomes are often mutually reinforcing.

Philosophically this sounds positive, but it also sets the bar higher for many substance users – it is no longer enough to be substance-free or to have controlled use of substances or access to safer substance using methods – that will no longer constitute success. Now one must also be a *productive member of society* and *personally fulfilled*. It is unclear what such an agenda might mean for harm reduction or the libertarian right to take risks and use substances; thus while the words with regard to a holistic agenda of treatment may sound inspiring, in a world of economic downturn, of known structural impacts and effects of substance use on the poorest, BME communities and vulnerable groups and at a time of budget cuts and PbR it might also give one pause for thought. There is evidence that social policies may be constructed to meet certain ends, but can end up having very different impacts, for example ASBOs and previous drug policies and youth justice policies (Measham and Moore 2008; Arnull 2013a); it is for this reason that there is a feeling of caution about what the new direction might bring.

Medications in Recovery (Strang 2012) is a wordy document which offers examples of what commissioning and treatment might look like in the new system and this is relevant to specialist practitioners. As a generic practitioner it will be accessible and intelligible, as much of what is suggested sounds like good, effective, holistic practice, which research about effective practice generally indicates is most effective when – it is individualised, specific about what the issues are, what is proposed as an intervention and why, and it is agreed with the service user what 'good' outcomes might look like and how one would know when they were achieved (see for example Fox and Arnull 2013).

A summary of the essential ingredients of what *Medications in Recovery* suggests a treatment service landscape that was recovery orientated would look like is below; this is not all verbatim, although some is:

> *A clear and coherent vision and framework for recovery visible to people in treatment, owned by all staff and maintained by strong clinical leadership:*
> * *For example does the service get involved in building communities of recovery that overlap with treatment, advocating for mutual aid, utilising peer supporters, ensuring recovery is visible to service users?*
>
> *Purposeful treatment interventions that are properly assessed, planned, measured, reviewed and adapted:*
> * *For example are assessment, planning, review and optimisation processes arranged so that treatment is active, individualised, and based on a proper understanding (and regular reviews) of an individual's changing problems, needs and strengths?*
>
> *'Phased and layered' interventions that reflect the different needs of people at different times:*
> * *For example developing phasing and layering interventions so that help appropriate to an individual's stage of recovery is available.*
> * *A range of treatment interventions available to meet needs of a range of clients including those with more complex needs.*
>
> *Treatment that creates the therapeutic conditions and optimism in which the challenge of initiating and maintaining change can be met, especially by those with few internal and external resources:*

- *For example, managers ensure keyworkers understand how and when to use a range of techniques and tools, including goal setting, empathetic listening, exploring the impact and negative consequences of current behaviour and the benefits of change, strategic use of problem recognition to amplify ambivalence about the status quo, managing rewards and negative contingencies, and involving social networks.*

Opiate Substitute Treatment programmes that optimise the medication aspect of the treatment according to the evidence and guidance:
- *For example audits to ensure:*
  - *Effective doses of OST are being prescribed as recommended in clinical guidance and tailored to the individual.*
  - *Supervised consumption is used as recommended*

Recovery measured by assessing and tracking improvements in severity, complexity and recovery capital. Use of this information to tailor interventions and support:
- *For example is progress regularly measured, and responded to, through intelligent use of the Treatment Outcomes Profile (TOP), drug testing, and measures of dependence, change motivation and engagement, skills and participation, environment, personality and relationships, risk and safeguarding, financial support, etc?*

Drug treatment not expected to deliver recovery on its own but integrated with and benefiting from other support such as mutual aid, employment support and housing:
- *For example has the service developed partnerships, joint working protocols and other ways of working with others able to provide recovery support, including mental health, employment, housing, mutual aid, recovery communities?*

Drug treatment – alongside peers and families – that provides direct access, sign-posts and or facilitated support to opportunities for reducing and stopping drug use, improving physical and mental health, engaging with others in recovery, improving relationships (including with children), finding meaningful work, building key life skills, and securing housing:
- *For example are arrangements in place for access to a broad range of recovery supports?*

(Strang 2012: 9)

As you can see there is nothing fundamentally 'new' about the recovery approach, it is simply a new focus on holistic support and recovery which aims to assist people to make changes right across their lives. With regard to the outgoing Models of Care (NTA 2006) language of tiers, it is worth generic practitioners understanding the language and model as it will apply to many commissioned treatment services for some time (depending on the commissioning cycle) and the language will still be common among specialist practitioners. However, services are now being commissioned to meet the conceptions of recovery informed methods of treatment, influenced by the language of 'layers' and 'phases' and driven by commissioning models that are treatment focused and directly or indirectly affected by PbR.

The language of 'tiers' made it easy to conceptualise the level of possible need/harm, what might be needed to effect change and offered a model on which to base a discussion with the service user, their family or relevant others (where appropriate) and other profession-als (again where appropriate). It was therefore simple and intelligible to many and had a defined and shared terminology; however, like other changes in the health and social care world during the late 1990s and early 2000s it was also believed to have became bureau-cratic and constraining (see NTA 2006; and other areas for example social work, Munro 2011; and academic discussion Saenz and Ugarte 2012). The hope is that by returning to more discretionary based work and by removing that level of prescription it may lead to greater flexibility.

The tiers of assessment looked like this:

Tier level	Type of intervention or treatment in this tier	Type of intervention or treatment in this tier	Type of intervention or treatment in this tier	Services based in prison should cover all of the tiers
Tier 1	Education and prevention: for example Life Education	Housing advice: provision for example that might provide access to supported accommodation for substance users	In-patient hepatology units – providing specialist hepatitis support which is generic	
Tier 2	Open access substance service: for example a drop in service	Drug Intervention Programme: enhanced Tier 2 access, for example arrest referral type schemes (DIP programmes can go across all levels)	Harm minimisation services: for example needle exchanges	
Tier 3	Structured assessment and care plan/ community-based services: for example a day programme	Methadone or any substitute prescription as part of a treatment programme	Brief intervention therapy – high level of contact and planning	
Tier 4	Detoxification – for example this may be in-patient or at home and overseen by the GP	Rehabilitation – therapeutic community – requiring at least 8 months in treatment	Structured Programme as part of a community-based court order	

As you can see all of these services remain relevant in a landscape of 'recovery'.

EXERCISE

Now copy the table and read *Models of Care – Updated 2006* – www.nta.nhs.uk/uploads/nta_modelsofcare_update_2006_moc3.pdf

Also download and read *Medications in Recovery* –

http://socialwelfare.bl.uk/subject-areas/services-activity/substance-misuse/nhs-nationaltreatmentagencyforsubstancemisuse/145798medications-in-recovery-main-report3.pdf

Add to the table, mapping the layers of service against the tiers you had already identified were available in your area: what might be the differences? How might this affect the services available? What might be the gains and losses? If possible, have a brief conversation with your local DAT or substance use treatment practitioners – what do they foresee?

Treatment and effectiveness

Treatment has been consistently shown to have some effect and this is particularly related to the first six years of treatment when the greatest gains are made (UKDPC 2012; EMCDDA 2012a; NTA 2012). Treatment has an immediate effect and that is most effectively maintained when the person remains in contact with the service for at least three months (NTA 2013; UKDPC 2012; EMCDDA 2012a; Arnull et al. 2007; Marsh and Cao 2005).

There are numerous treatment options and approaches which we shall discuss below, but what appears to be a fair, overall generalisation is that most forms of treatment work for some people in some circumstance when they are seeking help and support and this can have real health benefits and result in lifestyle changes for the substance user as a result of the therapeutic relationship. It is suggested that treatment is most effective when it is holistic – thus it addresses all of the needs of the service user, not just those immediately drug-related (NTA 2013; EMCDDA 2012a). This idea would be immediately accessible to most generic practitioners within the health and social care settings and the criminal and youth justice systems – thus not just substitute prescribing, but perhaps housing advice, counselling for underlying anxiety or past trauma, educational or work engagement when the person is at that stage, diversionary activity, health advice, support repairing family relationships or bonds, etc. However, what the NTA (2006) also had to say was that:

> While much of the focus of outcome research has been on identifying key individual characteristics that predict better treatment outcomes, such as higher levels of personal and social capital and lower levels of problem severity, increasing attention is being paid to service characteristics that can improve outcomes. The National Drug Evidence Centre research (2004) for the NTA showed that the best predictor of retention in community treatments in the north-west of England was related to service factors rather than client characteristics. Similarly, Meier (2005) has also reported that much of the variability in retention in residential rehabilitation services derives from the service itself rather than the service user. This is consistent with empirical research conducted in the US, which shows that organisational development work can lead to significantly enhanced treatment outcomes across patient populations.

Again this is further supported by the findings from the CTDM pilots (Arnull et al. 2007).

Reducing harm and introducing control

The range of theory and practice/intervention models under this umbrella is wide and covers all of the tiers of intervention. They range from highly theorised and researched models of intervention to generic services; we will consider each in more detail and look at some of the research that has underpinned or commented upon their effectiveness.

Educational, health, social care or generic service provision

Health advice and education by the state, charitable and private organisations and the media is usually conducted via campaigns and educational inputs. There are numerous examples and models, for example messages on cigarette packets and bottles of alcohol, and these are often the subject of fierce debate, for example recent debates about plain packaging and cigarettes in the UK (Channel 4 News 2013; Stirling University News 2013). Additionally, telephone helpline services, such as FRANK, aimed to meet a need for anonymised, factual information, advice and signposting, and other more generic services, such as ChildLine, can as we have seen, be the source of information and support.

Health advice and generic interventions may also be aimed at minimising harm, eg the minimum unit price for alcohol discussed in Chapter 4 and some of the work of Drinkaware, which seeks to promote positive drinking images about 'sensible' use.

Additionally, many educational programmes are delivered in school: for example the Life Education Programme, which is delivered on a national basis by Coram reaches 4,000 primary schools and involves 800,000 children. The Life Education Programme has been the subject of a considerable amount of research including an early RCT, which appeared to show no, or a small negative effect (Hawthorne et al. 1996), and many subsequent reviews and a recent systematic literature review have demonstrated effectiveness in raising children's awareness of their bodies and the effects of the environment and substances, including medicines, on them (Foxcroft et al. 2011; Faggiano et al. 2005; Ives et al. 2004). What remains unclear is how this subsequently affects substance trying or use; thus for example while there is no evidence of a causal link (this would be simply too complex to investigate given the sheer number of variables involved), we have seen sustained falls in drug trying and drug use during the period that we have had mandatory, universal substance use awareness education within schools (EMCDDA 2012b; UKDPC 2012). UKDPC (2012) argue that as universal preventative education is *inexpensive* and may have only a *very small positive effect*, it is nonetheless probably *cost-effective* and furthermore, that where general risk-taking type behaviour is targeted it may *impact on many kinds of risky behaviours, thus multiplying effects* (UKDPC 2012: 111).

Some form of substance use education has been mandatory as part of the national curriculum, although it is unclear how the deregulation of education undertaken by the coalition government will affect this. There are also specific educational programmes delivered within the CJS to offenders in the community and in prisons; for example it is possible if convicted of a drink driving offence to opt for a drink drive rehabilitation course, which if successfully completed allows the person to apply for their licence back at an earlier stage.[9]

Harm reduction approaches usually involve a designated part of treatment and intervention service with specialist workers who also have interest in areas such as sex work, body builders or gay or bisexual service users. Harm reduction services may involve needle exchanges, condoms, safe injecting equipment, etc.; they may also offer medical checks and health-based treatments, for example for abscesses.

ASBOs are a generic intervention used with frequency against substance users; they are aimed at limiting, curtailing or extinguishing certain behaviours and not at treatment (Fox and Arnull 2013). They may seek to limit public behaviours, such as drinking and shouting in the street, street-based injecting or allowing other people to use in your property or take substances, which may also affect your tenancy. We have discussed this form of social control of substance users at length in Chapter 5; as an approach it has been widely adopted by LAs (Measham and Moore 2008).[10]

Generic, wide-ranging family support services such as Sure Start (Eisenstadt 2013), Children's Centres and the Troubled Families Agenda (Department for Communities and Local Government), while not existing just to work with drug users are interventions that have targeted families where problematic or dependent use existed; as such they are based on a structural, social model of substance use and seek to support and build the whole family – this is the kind of work the EMCDDA (2012b) has indicated is successful. Family-based services, and in particular more intensive Family Therapy Services have also been found to be particular effective (NTA 2006).

Drop-in services are run by many specialist treatment services and aim to provide a place for people to seek advice, information and signposting that offers a 'face' and perhaps a community. Some service users will use drop-in services on a regular or frequent basis for a considerable period of time before they engage in treatment or interaction with harm minimisation services.

There are numerous services aimed generically at young people, which include substance awareness sessions, information, advice and signposting; these have improved significantly over the years as young people fed back that they wanted realistic, factual information and not 'scare tactics' (UKDPC 2012: 111). There are few services that aim at other particular groups of service users, such as women, BME groups, the elderly or those with learning disabilities – those which exist are often small, localised and based in the voluntary sector.

[9] Further information from the DVLA can be found at: www.direct.gov.uk/prod_consum_dg/groups/dg_digitalassets/@dg/@en/@motor/documents/digitalasset/dg_179001.pdf. If you search generally under this area you will find numerous private organisations offering advice, legal advice and representation, courses and information, etc. – this is both interesting and instructive as it suggests that there is a large number of people for whom this is relevant.

[10] A simple search will bring up numerous news reports related to this – for example www.mansfield.gov.uk/index.aspx?articleid=2443 and www.bournemouthecho.co.uk/news/9997283.Drug_dealers_given_ASBOs_to_keep_them_off_streets_of_Boscombe. This area is covered in the final chapter with a full exercise.

Abstinence-based programmes or treatment

These essentially cross all levels, 'tiers' or 'layers' of treatment and include:

- AA;
- NA;
- Families Anonymous;
- 12-step Minnesota Model programmes.

AA and NA approaches are discussed in more detail below.

Detoxification services may involve stabilising, assessing and then detoxifying a patient in a specialist facility, as an in-patient in a psychiatric wing or in the community supervised by a treatment agency and/or a GP. Research indicates that the former is the most effective (NTA 2006) and in my experience of working with substance users it was most effective when followed up by intensive, specialised support and treatment, preferably in a therapeutic community. However, some people may not wish to access this; detoxification may offer them some respite from drug use and help them to stabilise other health conditions. Drug overdose and death are, however, serious risks when someone is released from treatment and this is a period when people require planned support. The deaths of Amy Winehouse and Cory Monteith, the *Glee* star, were both reportedly shortly after they had undergone detoxification and perhaps some rehabilitation (*The Independent*, 8 January 2013 and BBC News, 17 July 2013).

Rehabilitation usually refers to in-patient, therapeutic communities. These are expensive and can be difficult to access; I personally spent a considerable amount of time working with people to complete numerous forms and stages of assessment before they would even learn whether they might be supported for treatment; this can be very stressful and quite a heartbreaking process when someone has reached the stage of being quite sure they need this level of support and treatment and are ready to make the commitment. This is an area where structural advantage clearly has benefits; if you are wealthy and can pay for your own treatment (or someone else can pay privately for you) then it is much easier to access. Rehabilitation used to often demand that people were drug- and alcohol-free on entry and that they achieved this by themselves; this has altered as part of the many changes we have seen effected within the treatment sector.

The evidence does indicate the effectiveness of rehabilitation programmes eight months or longer, especially when supported by appropriate aftercare services (NTA 2006); however, it should also be remembered that most 'ordinary' service users will not access or be able to access rehabilitation services until after many years of use and other forms of treatment and intervention, and as we know, it takes time and often many years for people to leave problematic or dependent use behind them. Amy Winehouse appears to have detoxified, but not to have considered she needed rehabilitative help[11] – the prognosis of the outcome in cases like this is often poor (NTA 2006).

[11] www.independent.co.uk/arts-entertainment/music/news/i-dont-want-to-die-amy-winehouses-words-just-hours-before-her-death-8442698.html, accessed 4 September 2013. The words of her song, 'I don't want to go to Rehab', sum up some of the issues and debates for substance users about choosing treatment or not.

Other forms of intervention where the service user is not at liberty include specialist wings in prison and in-patient psychiatric treatment; we have discussed both in some detail earlier in the book – see above and discussion in previous chapter.

'Self-help' services are dominated by AA and NA and for this reason we will cover them in some depth. Many meetings take place in premises that also belong to substance use treatment services. Those who attend may have stopped drinking or drug use and be abstinent – they may continue to attend meetings for many years or their whole lives. They may include those who are just beginning to consider that their use of substances is problematic and something they need to deal with; they may attend a meeting and continue to go; they may attend and go regularly thereafter; they may attend and find the service a stepping stone to other approaches that work better for them. In between those who have been involved in AA or NA for a long time and those who are just beginning are people who cover a whole range of positions between those two. AA and NA meetings attract many people from a range of social, class, race, gender[12] and other backgrounds and over the years AA and NA have adapted an insistence on a 'higher power' or 'god' in response to the breadth of their fellowship.

Although AA is essentially a user-led service it is a 12-step programme aligned to the Minnesota Model of Addiction (therefore usually denoted as Tiers 3 and 4). It was established in the USA during the 1930s and by 1946 the Twelve Traditions of Alcoholics Anonymous had been established. AA and NA are easily contacted via internet searches and what AA for example says about itself is this:

> *The Twelve Steps of Alcoholics Anonymous*
>
> *In simplest form, the AA program operates when a recovered alcoholic passes along the story of his or her own problem drinking, describes the sobriety he or she has found in AA, and invites the newcomer to join the informal Fellowship.*
>
> *The heart of the suggested program of personal recovery is contained in Twelve Steps describing the experience of the earliest members of the Society:*
>
> 1. *We admitted we were powerless over alcohol – that our lives had become unmanageable.*
> 2. *Came to believe that a Power greater than ourselves could restore us to sanity.*
> 3. *Made a decision to turn our will and our lives over to the care of God as we understood Him.*
> 4. *Made a searching and fearless moral inventory of ourselves.*
> 5. *Admitted to God, to ourselves and to another human being the exact nature of our wrongs.*
> 6. *Were entirely ready to have God remove all these defects of character.*
> 7. *Humbly asked Him to remove our shortcomings.*

[12] As we have seen, there are indications that this form of treatment and support is more successful for men and/or those whose alcohol use is related to social activity and ties.

8. *Made a list of all persons we had harmed, and became willing to make amends to them all.*
9. *Made direct amends to such people wherever possible, except when to do so would injure them or others.*
10. *Continued to take personal inventory and when we were wrong promptly admitted it.*
11. *Sought through prayer and meditation to improve our conscious contact with God as we understood Him, praying only for knowledge of His will for us and the power to carry that out.*
12. *Having had a spiritual awakening as the result of these steps, we tried to carry this message to alcoholics and to practice these principles in all our affairs.*

Newcomers are not asked to accept or follow these Twelve Steps in their entirety if they feel unwilling or unable to do so.

They will usually be asked to keep an open mind, to attend meetings at which recovered alcoholics describe their personal experiences in achieving sobriety, and to read AA literature describing and interpreting the AA program.

AA members will usually emphasize to newcomers that only problem drinkers themselves, individually, can determine whether or not they are in fact alcoholics.

As you will see, the AA programme draws on concepts of disease, considering alcohol dependence as a *malady of the emotions, mind and body*; it endorses concepts of addiction, loss of control or will, spirituality and fellowship; for many people it is helpful, including celebrities, such as Russell Brand, who talk openly about how concepts similar to those espoused by AA have been useful to them. However, AA itself seeks anonymity both at a personal, group and organisational level – it describes its marketing strategy as one aimed at *attracting* rather than promoting and within the UK there are currently about 4,400 groups that meet and approximately 2 million fellows or members.[13] AA's literature is accessible and easy to read and it is clear about its value base and treatment approach.

Hard 'evidence' about AA and NA approaches is less easy to come by in part because of the anonymity of the approach and because there have been few research exercises able to discount other variables and thus 'prove' that it was *this* intervention that made a difference. The range of studies appears to suggest that at worst AA/NA do no harm and may be more effective than no intervention and may be as effective as other treatment approaches including cognitive behavioural therapy (CBT) (Arkowitz and Lilienfeld 2011). However, critics argue that it can also be fanatical, critical, judging and hostile to those who do not accept all of its tenets; Chris Owen, writing in the *Independent* on 1 February 2013 reported his own and others' experiences. What Owen and others appear to struggle with is the almost religious zeal and surrender that AA and NA approaches can be seen to espouse, which is now less commonly and widely accepted in many European countries and cultures:

---

[13] Taken from the AA website – www.alcoholics-anonymous.org.uk/About-AA/AA-Structure-in-Great-Britain, accessed 22 July 2013.

> *AA tells you it is the only way to stay sober, fall from the path and you will relapse, and it is this, coupled with the focus on aggrandising the addiction beyond all proportion into an unbeatable foe, a demon you cannot defeat, only keep a constant watch on, that grates.*[14]

Owen (2013) also suggests there is estrangement from other users and denigration of other approaches if the tenets are questioned in any way.

An RCT reported by Kelly and Hoeppner (2013) indicated that it was not the 12-steps that appeared linked to treatment success but the lessening of pro-social drinking ties through the creation of a new social group that was pro-abstinence (although this effect was less strong). Drawing on a matched comparison sample group trial, which was reported widely ('Project Match' undertaken in the USA), Kelly and Hoeppner (2013) considered the impact of gender on the AA approach and found that gender had a mediating effect.

They suggested that the lessening of the pro-social drinking ties may have accounted for this differential effect as this was less strongly associated with women's drinking. The importance of the findings seem to be therefore that 12-step and AA/NA type approaches can offer support to some people who are open to them. The model appears to support some in certain circumstances but those effects can be differentially felt and this may be mediated by gender as a result of the particular treatment effect which AA appears to possess, namely the loosening of pro-social drinking networks. It is therefore important to consider with a service user the nature of their drinking and to understand whether or not this may be a factor that has relevance for them; for example this approach may or may not be relevant to some users from particular ethnic or cultural backgrounds where their alcohol use is hidden or already 'frowned upon' and thus does not form part of their social behaviour.

Specialist, structured substance use treatment

Treatment for service users draws on a range of therapeutic approaches and keyworking relationships. The NTA defined good practice within a keyworking relationship as requiring the following elements:

- Following triage/assessment, drawing up an initial care plan if required to address immediate needs (eg providing information and advice on drug and alcohol misuse).
- Harm reduction interventions.
- Motivational interventions to enhance retention.
- Developing and agreeing the care plan with the client and ensuring implementation of the care plan – with interventions relevant to each stage of the treatment journey and regular care plan reviews. (NTA 2006: 45)

The NTA (2006) then went on to describe a range of interventions they grouped together and described as *evidence-based psychosocial interventions*:

[14] Chris Owen, *The Independent*, 1 February 2013 – www.independent.co.uk/voices/comment/alcoholics-anonymous-do-extraordinary-brave-work-for-people-who-are-in-need-but-my-journey-to-sobriety-shows-their-technique-isnt-for-everyone-8477252.html

- CBT;

- coping skills training;

- relapse prevention therapy;

- motivational interventions;

- contingency management;

- community reinforcement approaches;

- some family approaches.

They qualified this by saying that psychosocial interventions needed to follow assessment and be structured and planned and preferably *delivered by a demonstrably competent practitioner* (NTA 2006: 44)

We will consider two of the most common approaches briefly, CBT and MI.

CBT

CBT is an approach that has been widely adopted within the criminal justice and prison-based systems in part as a result of the proselytising of psychologists within the prison system and because they were able to 'evidence' their effectiveness at a time when other treatments and therapies were less able to do so (see discussion in Fox and Arnull 2013: 63–7 and also Paylor et al. 2012). CBT approaches are well known to many professional groups and practitioners and may therefore feel accessible (Paylor et al. 2012: 67 concerning social workers). They are an intervention approved by NICE as a 'talking therapy of choice' and are derived from social learning theory. CBT is concerned with conscious thought and is based on the idea that we behave in a way we have learned or been conditioned to; using the therapeutic process *it seeks to alter the cognitive processes and effect change* (Fox and Arnull 2013: 65). CBT uses terms such as 'modelling appropriate behaviour', 'positively reinforcing' acceptable behaviour and 'extinguishing' inappropriate or unacceptable behaviour. It can be delivered on an individual or group basis. Effectiveness has been shown to be greatest when the intervention is delivered by a qualified practitioner. Critiques of CBT are that is not necessarily open about seeking to change the way the service user thinks. Furthermore, that exponents of CBT extol its virtues and effectiveness, but when it does not demonstrate an 'effect' they 'blame' a lack of programme integrity, effectiveness of the worker(s) or some other variable, rather than question the method or its appropriateness in that instance, or that effectiveness may be less than that claimed.

Motivational interviewing

Motivational interviewing has become very popular within substance treatment services. I trained in MI and received regular clinical supervision paid for by the probation service in the mid-1990s. At that time it was quite new in the UK, not widely used and was in many ways quite distinct from some of the interpretations I see discussed and practised today; it has therefore become a wide 'brand', much as CBT, and incorporates a whole range of approaches. My training and knowledge of MI was very much related to the Transtheoretical

Model, which was put forward by Prochaska and diClemente (1982, 1998); the cycle of change and the treatment philosophy and approach were subtly different from what many now refer to as the 'wheel of change' model (Goodman 2007). The work of Prochaska and diClemente proposed that behaviour went through or could be mapped against a series of steps when an individual was considering change. This might lead us on occasions to 'advance' or on other occasions to make no move or to move forward and then fall back – for many people who had sought to make changes in their lives at some point the model had some resonance. What they suggested was that the model could be used to help people who were substance dependent or engaged in other 'addictive' behaviours to understand their behaviour, make and sustain change.

The model included stages such as:

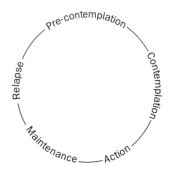

The cycle was originally drawn as a circle, which I found helpful and still do; the many people I worked with using this model also thought so. You could enter the cycle at any point for a range of different behaviours and you could move backwards or forwards across any of the stages – contemplation was seen as a very uncomfortable (and therefore quite often risky) place for anyone to be.

One of the things I loved about MI and that drew me to it as a practitioner was the control it gave to the service user; the ability for them to work openly and explicitly with you about where they saw themselves in relation to a range of issues they might wish to address, or others might wish them to address (remember I was a probation officer and thus the service user had given a legal undertaking to the court to think about change and their offending behaviour as part of their order or licence). I found the model very accessible to many service users as it could easily be diagrammatically displayed and most people could relate different aspects of their lives to it. Differently from how it is sometimes reported, therefore, I considered the approach gave control to the service user; if substance use appeared to be problematic in their lives (ie they had health problems or their offending related to substance use) but they did not consider this problematic I would have regarded it unethical to work to 'jog' or 'move' them from pre-contemplation to contemplation without being quite explicit that I wanted to consider that part of the cycle. It was important to work with them on why they were quite sure there was no issue, when others, for example the court or family members, might say otherwise. The techniques are complex and involve a number of areas of behaviour and self-concept and thus require serious consideration of how you work with people in terms of self-esteem for example. Working on self-esteem can be problematic if this is an area in which the person has considerable value linked to the problematic behaviour – eg drug taking or injecting – thus, use of the method in any detail requires significant training and clinical supervision, as the NTA (2006) outline. As a method simply of engaging someone in a discussion of their behaviour it is a valuable means to do so and it appears this is the way it is most commonly used and understood in many areas of generic practice and within Tier 2 or keyworking relationships in substance use treatment services. It has been shown to be most effective as a method of intervention when used by trained specialist practitioners (NTA 2006).

Because there has been so much interest in MI and the Cycle of Change there have been numerous reviews of its effectiveness and these have included systematic reviews and some RCTs. The evidence remains disputed, some approaches have shown little or no effect and others have shown more effectiveness than other therapeutic methods. In general, like the other treatment approaches considered so far it has not usually been seen to be harmful and in general to have been more helpful than not – thus Wanigarante et al. (2005) suggested MI was especially effective when combined with brief interventions, whereas Lai et al. (2010) found the approach to be no more or less effective than other approaches such as individual counselling. Critiques of MI are that it is an approach which has been 'bastardised' and thus like some CBT designated interventions it is not always clear how much integrity there has been to the care plan or the treatment method. It is an approach recommended by the NTA (2006) who, as we have seen, have drawn attention to the importance of service delivery factors and thus the impact this may or may not have on the effectiveness of the methods of intervention.

A meta-analytic review by Jensen et al. (2011: 433) found a *small, but significant post treatment effect* as the result of MI interventions with adolescents; they concluded strongly that these *were effective across a variety of substance use behaviours, varying session lengths and different settings and for interventions that used clinicians with different levels of education*. Their findings were therefore more significant and positive than some of those reported for adults; this suggests that MI is an intervention type worth considering for young people for whom substance dependency/problematic use is an issue.

Interventions are also delivered via the CJS and via the mental health system as we have seen. They contain many elements of the treatment approaches discussed above and may cross all four tiers. Interventions within the CJS have been heavily researched post-1998 and in general, treatment effectiveness is indicated both in lowering problematic substance use and offending behaviour (see for example Department of Health 1996; Gossop 2005; NTA 2006).

An initial assessment toolkit

This basic assessment toolkit seeks to outline how assessment skills can be utilised by all as generic practitioners to undertake an initial assessment of a drug or alcohol user and their family. It seeks to enable this in a way that is explicit and inclusive, encouraging the sharing and thinking through of needs, issues and options and decisions about where, when or if more specialist advice is required and if so from whom, when and how.

What is the area of concern?	Why is this area of concern?	Who considers this to be of concern and what actions have they taken?	Change/action required and by whom – has this person agreed to this or to consider this?	Treatment required and why? Who will provide the treatment?
For example:				
Alcohol use	Drunk every weekend night; comes home arguing, shouting and being verbally threatening to wife	Neighbours who have called police Wife who has sought counselling from her GP, discussed the matter with family and close friends and sought legal advice regarding a separation	Joe, to lower the amount of evenings he goes out drinking – Yes Joe says committed Joe to lower the amount he drinks – Yes says he is committed Joe to begin to think about what happens when he drinks to excess – Joe doesn't think there is a problem – he thinks people exaggerate and wind him up. Mary and Joe to think about whether they might socialise together and in a different environment than the pub – Yes both agree to this Mary to think about what steps she wishes to take and what help she may need to take those steps, for example more legal advice etc. – no intervention – Mary wishes to just think about this on her own	Information giving re the effects of alcohol on the body and brain. Local alcohol service Information giving re excessive drinking and the effects of alcohol and the family – local alcohol service Joe and Mary to think about next steps – would either of them like to access family therapy, couple therapy or Joe alcohol counselling or a treatment/intervention. Proposed – GP counsellor for two initial joint sessions Mary to consider single session with GP counsellor or Family Support Worker at local alcohol service
Other issues/ questions practitioner may have…	Are there any safeguarding or domestic violence concerns? Are there any monetary concerns because of the level of alcohol use? Are there any you might have in addition?			

Concluding thoughts

The treatment scene is currently in flux – it is moving from a time of 'tiers' to 'layers' and 'phases' of treatment; however, these are not really so different from what good practice and research-based practice has demonstrated is most effective – that treatment approaches should be person-centred and inclusive, they should work with the service user to think about their whole life and be explicit about what will be done, when, by whom, in what circumstances and when and how it would be known that the outcomes had been achieved.

The notions of recovery are congruent with a holistic, social model of substance use. The commissioning of services will be affected by this change and thus by an apparent lowering of focus on process and treatment types and more of a focus on outcomes. However, it would seem that there is some inherent conflict within the system: PbR schemes will pay when the service user is substance-free at a six-month follow-up stage, but *Medications in Recovery* (NTA 2012) suggests no 'arbitrary limits' should be set (specifically with regard to substitute prescribing) but infused as an argument throughout the whole. Additionally, while the PbR pilot and evaluation have not yet been completed many services are being commissioned on the basis of outcomes and performance.[15]

The coalition government's localism agenda (which is also infused in the *Medications in Recovery* document) presents a move away from centralised advice and support; this is further underlined by the removal of the NTA and regional teams and their replacement with LA-based responsibility for public health and a national body (for example within England it is PHE) providing coverage on issues of national importance, and some overall structure and guidance. Clearly this is an emerging picture as the policy framework only came into place in April 2013, but it suggests the potential for innovation and local difference, but also for fragmentation and the loss of expertise; furthermore there are concerns that it may in the future be harder to evidence substance use and outcomes and comparable regional and local performance, funding and input. These sorts of arguments and effects are already being made and witnessed in other social policy areas, for example within the YJS.[16]

It cannot be known at this time what the impact of these changes will be; what remains constant is that drug policy in particular reflects the sea changes in more general social policy – in this case localism, increased discretion, privatisation, a move away from monitored and supported effective practice guidance and towards overarching, loosely structured guidance. Drug policy has since 1995 been fast-paced and ever changing and this presents challenges for the student and the generic practitioner. Alcohol policy is more emergent – it appears to be following the moral trajectories of drug policy but to be the subject of significant influence as the result of business concerns about the impact of proposed changes, for example unit pricing. The drinks industry is a powerful lobby and provides much work and export income for certain sectors of the UK; should illicit drug use be legalised it is to be anticipated the impact would then be similar.

[15] Anecdotal reports.
[16] Anecdotal reports.

Within the treatment sphere many things will remain much the same in a wider context of commissioning changes and the structure of provision. The language and expectations underpinning treatment, commissioning and provision will be familiar to many and they will include features to be found elsewhere across the health and social policy field in the foreseeable future. For substance users it is unclear where the current focus on 'recovery' will lead – it may hold within itself the potential for unintended outcomes, which may have negative effects, although *Medications in Recovery* (Strang 2012) and Hayes (NTA 2013) have spoken with hope of its possibilities for delivering treatment and care that is person-centred and holistic. As we have seen, drug and alcohol policy have not always had the effects intended (Arnull 2013a) and some of the effects have been negative and stigmatising in the way they have impacted policy and treatment. In other areas, such as criminal justice, there were many concerns that there would be negative impacts and yet there appear to have been many beneficial effects for treatment services and substance users (NTA 2013). Predicting or foretelling policy outcomes is not easy, and in the area of substance use where the mix of emotion and opinion is ever present, alongside a powerful and contradictory international agenda, it is even less straightforward.

7 Values

Introduction

This short chapter builds on work undertaken throughout the book, which seeks to engage the reader in a series of exercises and case studies that focus on values. As discussed, the intention is to enable the reader to think critically and reflectively about how values are formed and how this affects the perspective taken with regard to substance use and the way substance users are responded to. The exercises throughout the book allow the reader to explore their unspoken and unacknowledged attitudes that affect their values.

The intention is that the reader will be able to reflect upon and understand where their own values come from and thus be enabled to use theory to write about it and incorporate it critically into their own thinking and/or practice where this is applicable. There is emerging evidence that reflective learning enables practitioners to work in an anti-oppressive way because they are better equipped as independent, critical thinkers and practitioners and thus potentially *in a better position to reflect upon planned or sudden change and, through their reflection and to offer appropriate and considered professional challenge* (Arnull and Aldridge-Bent 2013). Learning in a reflective way can help to develop an inner, but conscious and critical dialogue between theory and practice and thus encourage a dialectical process. In addition, knowledge of self, gained through the previous chapters, can enable the reader to learn and practise in an evidence-based way – *consciously, explicitly and judiciously* (Sackett et al. 1996: 71).

This chapter is almost entirely exercise-based; it presents exercises you can undertake on your own and with others; it aims to extend your thinking and your reflection. The exercises in this chapter can be used as a teaching aid or resource.

Experiences of substance use

There are many people who have written about their own experiences of substance use and dependency – these include some we have already discussed such as Russell Brand (2008, 2013) and Chris Owen (*The Independent*, 1 February 2013). You can find your own sources or you might also consider *The Howard Marks Book of Dope Stories* (Marks 2002).

EXERCISE

Read at least one account and then reflect on:

» *What was your immediate reaction to what they wrote?*

» *How similar is their use, experience or knowledge of substances to your own? What is different, how and why?*

Sybille Bedford was a fiction writer who drew on her own life in her writing; this included living and coping with her mother's dependent use of morphine; you can read a brief biography of her at www.sybillebedford.com/life. The book about her experiences with her mother is called *Jigsaw: An Unsentimental Education – A Biographical Novel*.

EXERCISE

Read all or some of her account and then re-read the chapter concerning families and substance use and the effects on dependents, family members, children and young people. Have your ideas or views stayed the same? Does Sybille Bedford's experience help you to think about those issues in any way that is different? Explain your answer.

In addition, compare her coverage of her mother's growing dependence on what had originally been prescribed medication, to more recent news coverage of the use and abuse of prescribed medication – for example *The Sunday Times*, 8 September 2013, 'A Nation of Pill Poppers'.

EXERCISE

What do you think are the similarities between the issues and the accounts? How do you think these might be tackled? How do others suggest these might be tackled? Do you consider there is a difference between dependence on prescribed medication and dependence on alcohol or illicit substances? Account for your answer.

Effects of substance use

Drawing on the previous chapters, complete the table below; for a particular substance or group of substances in the first instance do so simply drawing on what you can recall. Then do so in a more systematic fashion, checking what you have written thus far for accuracy. Complete the table with particular reference to the practice field and geographical area in which you work, or your area of study.

Table adapted from UDPC report 2012

	Individual	Family	Friends and peers	Community	National	International
Harm to health						
Social harms						
Structural harms						
Economic harms						
Environmental harms						

Stigmatisation

As we have seen, one of the effects of substance use can be stigmatisation. Complete the following exercises, which are aimed to help you reflect upon this.

EXERCISE

» Drawing on the table above outline how in an area of your practice or learning stigmatisation might impact negatively on a substance user and/or their family. How might this be practically tackled? Outline three steps.

» You may also wish to read all or some of J. K. Rowling's The Casual Vacancy (2012), which in fictional form explores the issues of stigmatisation of drug users, the impact of this and a community's concerns about a treatment centre. Think about areas of practice you are familiar with or know about in the area you live or work: how might stigmatisation affect individuals, families and communities in that area, people that you know or with whom you have worked?

Moving away from your own areas of knowledge and practice consider now the wider social policy and theoretical issues we have discussed in earlier chapters. Refresh your memory of the issues you discussed there and the policy trajectories that followed and the impacts and outcomes it is argued those had.

Then read the article below[1] and search on the web for other similar news stories:

Mansfield District Council has been successfully granted an ASBO against an anti social, prolific drug user.

---

[1] www.mansfield.gov.uk/index.aspx?articleid=2443, accessed 4 September 2013.

[Full Name] (27), of Birch House, Vicars Court, Clipstone was made subject to an Anti-Social Behaviour Order by Mansfield Magistrates on 22 October after a series of threatening incidents involving drink and drugs in Mansfield Town Centre.

[note: here in the article a full face picture of the man is shown – this has been removed].

During the three month period between May and August this year, [Full Name] was observed taking drugs on six occasions. On one occasion he was caught on CCTV injecting his left arm at the rear of St John's Church.

[Full Name] had already been banned from Mansfield Library and the Four Seasons Centre after taking drugs in the toilets of both premises and being drunk on several occasions.

He had also been caught urinating against the wall of Iceland in the Rosemary Centre.

Under the terms of the Act, [Full Name] is banned from acting or threatening to act in a manner likely to cause harassment, alarm and distress to anyone in the District of Mansfield.

He is also banned from the following in Mansfield Town Centre:

- *Entering all retail premises, public toilets, churches and church grounds and the public library.*
- *Being drunk and disorderly.*
- *Carrying or consuming alcohol from an open container in public.*
- *Urinating in public.*
- *Possessing or using controlled drugs.*
- *Being verbally abusive to any person not of the same household as himself and in particular officers and agents of Mansfield District Council, PSCO's, Police Officers and Security Staff.*

Councillor Danny McCrossan, Portfolio Holder for Public Protection at Mansfield District Council, commented: 'I am pleased that this Anti-Social Behaviour Order has been granted.'

'This individual has undertaken a series of antisocial, threatening and intimidating acts in Mansfield Town Centre which could have placed members of the public in real danger.'

'The granting of this ASBO is an excellent example of the partnership between Mansfield District Council, Town Centre Shops, Mansfield Library and Notts Police working together to rid the town of such nuisance individuals. I hope this sends out a clear message that such behaviour will not be tolerated.'

Breach of an ASBO is a criminal offence. If you see [Full Name] breaking the terms of his ASBO contact Mansfield Police on 01623 420999.

EXERCISE

What do you think the possible impacts of such stories are? What might be the benefits and for whom? What might be the negative effects and for whom? Did social policy impact upon or create the circumstances in which this could happen? If so how?

Generic practitioners: using research – recognising and referring

In Chapter 5 we discussed the research by Gilbert et al. (2009), which argued that there was the possibility of better long-term outcomes for young people if emotional neglect and abuse are identified at an early stage. In the same chapter we also considered how substance use and dependency is often missed in work with older adults – this is a growing area of concern.

Gilbert et al. (2009) suggested that substance use generic practitioners could and should use validated assessment checklists more frequently as these could play an important role in enabling more effective assessment and identification of issues.

EXERCISE

Look up at least two validated assessment checklists from the link given in Chapter 5 (Cox and Bentovim 2000). Where and how might these be used in practice? Who might use them, when and why? If you are working in or have any practice experience in health and social care, can you think of any circumstances in which you could have used these checklists? If so detail your answer – when, how, why?

Planning reflective interventions

This tool was developed by me in 2011 as part of my teaching for newly qualified social workers; I have developed it further for use as part of the teaching process. I have also written about this tool and presented at the International Reflective Practice Conference in 2013 along with a colleague: 'Can learning tools help students practise and build theory-practice-reflection?' The tool is presented here but should not be reproduced without permission.

Exercise sheet: planning reflective interventions

Think about a recent piece of work or one you will be engaging with in the near future – answer the following:

- *Describe the situation.*
- *What are the main issues you need to be aware of in this piece of work from a practice perspective?*
- *What is the organisational context?*
- *What is the reason/justification/rationale for your involvement?*
- *What are your duties (legal and otherwise) here?*

- *What does your line manager/other manager/colleagues expect you to do?*

- *What does the client/service user anticipate?*

- *Do you have all of the information you need to proceed? If not – how/where/from whom are you going to get it? Within what timescale?*

- *What other professionals do you need to contact/liaise with?*

- *What theoretical perspective underpins your proposed method of intervention? How does this help? If you do not know, how/when are you going to find out?*

- *Have you looked at/considered recent relevant research into methods of intervention/ effectiveness/outcomes in this area? If yes, how has this helped? If not when/how will you do this?*

- *What outcomes are you anticipating/hoping for? Short and long-term.*

- *Is there anything that affects your empathy for this client/situation?*

- *Are there any value/AOP issues which you need to consider? Have you done this? What are the implications?*

- *Have you thought creatively about all options?*

- *What is your planned intervention ... If it does not yet exist how will you get it into place in time?*

- *How or with whom will you reflect on:*

    1. *the planning process;*
    2. *the intervention itself as a process;*
    3. *the theory;*
    4. *the method(s) used;*
    5. *the outcomes;*
    6. *values issues raised;*
    7. *the emotional responses of participants – you, client, others including professionals.*

Thinking about the proforma above, consider further the section regarding contact and work with other professionals – refresh yourself with regard to Chapters 2 and 3. How does your understanding of work with other professionals inform your understanding of the need for substance use policy to be based on partnership work and inter-professional practice?

Concluding remarks

The intention of the exercises is to help you to formulate and explore how your theoretical knowledge interacts with your or others' practice knowledge (where that is relevant) and how in turn these are both impacted by your own personal experience, knowledge, emotions and circumstances. The exercises are only as good as the energy, honesty and commitment you are able to put into them – they may be difficult, you may wish to ensure they are anonymised and kept private, you may wish to seek help, counselling or advice as a result of their completion – there are numerous confidential helplines and Alcohol Concern has a comprehensive list that can be accessed at: www.alcoholconcern.org.uk/links.

References

Advisory Council on the Misuse of Drugs (ACMD) (1971) *The Classification of Cannabis under the Misuse of Drugs Act 1971*. London: HMSO

Advisory Council on the Misuse of Drugs (ACMD) (1982) *Treatment and Rehabilitation*. London: HMSO

Advisory Council on the Misuse of Drugs (ACMD) (2003) *Hidden Harm: Responding to the Needs of Children of Problem Drug Users*. Report of an inquiry by the Advisory Council on the Misuse of Drugs. London: Home Office

Arkowitz, H. and Lilienfeld, S.O. (2011) 'Does Alcoholics Anonymous Work?' *Scientific American Mind* 22: 64–5. Published online: 17 February 2011. doi: 10.1038/scientificamericanmind0311-64

Armstrong, D., Cummings, C., Jones, K., and McConville, E. (2011) 'Welfare to Work Commissioning – Wave Two Provider Survey'. Research Report 757, Department for Work and Pensions. http://research.dwp.gov.uk/asd/asd5/rrs-index.asp, accessed 2 September 2013

Arnull, E. (2007) *The Development and Implementation of Drug Policy in England 1994–2004*. Published thesis. London: Middlesex University

Arnull, E. (2009) 'Drug Policy and Performance Management: A Necessary Evil?'. *Drugs: Education, Prevention and Policy* 16(4): 298–310

Arnull, E. (2013a) 'That's Not What I Meant ...': Unintended Effects and Policy Outcomes'. *Journal of Criminology and Social Integration* 21(1)

Arnull, E. (2013b) 'Care to Parent'. Unpublished report for Buckinghamshire County Council

Arnull, E. (2014) 'Social Work and the Youth Justice System: Ensuring Social Work Values'. *PROBATION Junior Journal*

Arnull, E. and Aldridge-Bent, S. (2013) 'Can learning tools help students practice and build theory-practice-reflection?' Paper given at the 17th International Reflective Practice Conference, Swansea, September

Arnull, E. and Eagle, S. (2009) *Girls offending: patterns, perceptions and interventions*. London: YJB

Arnull, E., Eagle, S., Patel, S. and Gammampila, A. (2007) *An Evaluation of the Crack Treatment Delivery Model*. London: Department of Health, NTA

Arsenault, L. Cannon, M., Witton, J. and Murray, R.M. (2004) 'Causal Association between Cannabis and Psychosis: Examination of the Evidence'. *British Journal of Psychiatry* 184: 110–17

Baker, P. (1991) 'Drug Advisory Committees in Practice: Disjointed Coordination'. *Druglink* 6(5): 12–13

Baker, P. and Runnicles, D. (1991) *Co-ordinating Drugs Services: The Role of Regional and District Drug Advisory Committees*. London: London Research Centre and Local Government Drugs Forum

Barnard, M. (2007) *Drug Addiction and Families*. London: Jessica Kingsley

BBC (21 May 2012) 'EU austerity drive country by country'. www.bbc.co.uk/news/10162176, accessed 2 September 2013

BBC (27 September 2012) 'Rochdale abuse: Social services "missed opportunities"'. www.bbc.co.uk/news/uk-england-manchester-19739073, accessed 2 September 2013

BBC (9 January 2013) 'Private sector rehabilitation plans defended by government'. www.bbc.co.uk/news/uk-20953644, accessed 2 September 2013

BBC (7 May 2013) 'Addict parents are "not all bad" says Tam Baillie'. www.bbc.co.uk/news/uk-scotland-22432274, accessed 2 September 2013

BBC (2 September 2013) Timeline of Baby P case. www.bbc.co.uk/news/uk-11626806, accessed 2 September 2013

BBC News (2013) 'The reclassification of cannabis'. http://news.bbc.co.uk/1/hi/7845023.stm, accessed 10 June 2013

BBC News (1 March 2013) 'Call for UK-wide 50p per unit price'. www.bbc.co.uk/news/health-21621144, accessed 10 April 2013

BBC News (27 June 2007) 'Brown is UK's new prime minister'. news.bbc.co.uk/1/hi/6245682.stm, accessed 2 April 2013

Bedford, S. (1989) *Jigsaw: An Unsentimental Education – A Biographical Novel*. London: Penguin

Bellew, R. (2012) *Coram Life Education: Evidence of Outcomes*. October. London: Coram

Bennett, T. (2001) 'Drugs and Crime – The Results of Research on Drugs Testing and Interviewing Arrestees'. Home Office Research Study 183

Berridge, V. (1996) *AIDS in the UK: The Making of Policy, 1981–1994*. Oxford: Oxford University Press

Berridge, V. (2007) *Marketing Health: Smoking and the Discourse of Public Health in Britain, 1945–2000*. Oxford: Oxford University Press

Berten, H., Cardoen, D., Brondeel, R. and Vettenburg, N. (2012) 'Alcohol and Cannabis Use among Adolescents in Flemish Secondary Schools in Brussels: Effects of Type of Education'. *BMC Public Health* 12: 215

Bierderman, J., Faraone, S.V., Monuteaux, M.C. and Feighner, J.A. (2000) 'Patterns of Alcohol and Drug Use in Adolescents can be Predicted by Parental Substance Use Disorders'. *Pediatrics* 106: 4792–7

Blunkett, D. (2006) *The Blunkett Tapes*. London: Bloomsbury

Bourgois, P. (2003) 'Crack and the Political Economy of Social Suffering'. *Addiction Research and Social Theory* 11(1): 31–7

Bourgois, P. (2008) 'The Mystery of Marijuana: Science and the U.S. War on Drugs'. *Substance Use & Misuse* 43: 581–3

Bourgois P., Martinez, A., Kral, A., Edlin, B.R. and Schonberg, J. (2006) 'Reinterpreting Ethnic Patterns among White and African American Men Who Inject Heroin: A Social Science of Medicine Approach'. *PLoS Med* 3(10): e452

Bourgois, P. and Schonberg, J. (2007) 'Intimate Apartheid: Ethnic Dimensions of Habitus among Homeless Heroin Injectors'. *Ethnography* 8(1): 7–32

Brand, R. (1998) *My Booky Wooky*. London: Hodder

Bremner, P., Burnett, J., Mistral, W., Nunney, F. and Ravat, M. (2011) *Young People, Alcohol and Their Influences*. York: Joseph Rowntree Foundation

British Association of Social Work (BASW) (2012) 'Code of Ethics for Social Work: Statement of Principles'. Birmingham: BASW

British Library (26 March 2013) 'Social Sciences Blog: "Addictive Personality": Myth or Reality?' http://britishlibrary. typepad.co.uk/socialscience/2013/03/addictive-personality-myth-or-reality.html, accessed 5 September 2013

Bronfenbrenner, U. (1994) 'Ecological Models of Human Development'. In *International Encyclopedia of Education*, Vol. 3. 2nd edition. Oxford: Elsevier

Brown, P. and Sparks, R. (eds) (1989) *Beyond Thatcherism: Social Policy, Politics and Society*. Milton Keynes: Open University Press

Buchanan, J. (2010) 'Drug Policy under New Labour 1997–2010: Prolonging the War on Drugs'. *Probation Journal* 57(3): 250–62

Cabinet Office Behavioural Insights Team (2010) *Applying Behavioural Insight to Health*. London: HMSO

Calafat, A., Kronegger, L., Juan, M., Duch, M.A. and Kosir, M. (2011) 'Influence of the Friends Network in Drug Use and Violent Behaviour among Young People in the Nightlife Recreational Context'. *Psicothema* 23: 544–51

Campbell, E. (2013) 'Transgression, Affect and Performance: Choreographing a Politics of Urban Space'. *British Journal of Criminology* 53(1): 18–40

Castree, A. (1995) 'The Role of the Police in Tackling Drugs Crime'. Drugs, Rights and Justice: Organised by Release as part of Liberty's Convention on Human Rights. www.drugscope.org.uk, accessed September 2004

Centre for Mental Health, DrugScope and UKDPC (2012) 'Dual Diagnosis: A Challenge for the Reformed NHS and Public Health England. A Discussion Paper from the Centre for Mental Health, DrugScope and the UKDPC'. www.drugscope.org.uk/Resources/Drugscope/Documents/PDF/Policy/DSDualDiagnosisDiscussionPaper.pdf, accessed 21 July 2013

Cheliotis, L.K. (2006) 'How Iron is the Iron Cage of New Penology? The Role of Human Agency in the Implementation of Criminal Justice Policy'. *Punishment & Society* 8: 313–40

Coram Life Education (2011) 'Evidence of Outcomes: Key Findings October 2011'. London: Coram

Cox, A. and Bentovim, A. (2000) *Framework for the Assessment of Children in Need and their Families: The Family Pack of Questionnaires and Scales*. London: Department of Health

Cusick, L. and Hickman, M. (2005) '"Trapping" in Drug Use and Sex Work Careers'. *Drugs: Education, Prevention and Policy* 12(5): 369–79. http://informahealthcare.com/doi/abs/10.1080/09687630500226779

Cusick, L., Martin, A. and May, T. (2003) *Vulnerability and Involvement in Drug Use and Sex Work*. Research Findings 247. London: Home Office

Dale-Perrera, A. (2001) 'National Treatment Agency: Building Castles on Sand'. *Druglink* 16(3): 19–21

Davies, J.S. (2002) 'Regeneration Partnerships under New Labour: A Case of Creeping Centralisation'. In C. Glendinning, M. Powell and K. Rummery (eds), *Partnerships, New Labour and the Governance of Welfare*. Bristol: Policy Press, 167–82

Davies, J.S. (2005) 'Local Governance and the Dialectics of Hierarchy, Market and Network'. *Policy Studies* 25(3/4): 311–35

Deacon, A. and Mann, K. (1999) 'Agency, Modernity and Social Policy'. *Journal of Social Policy* 28(3): 413–45

Deakin, N. (1994) *The Politics of Welfare: Continuities and Change*. Hemel Hempstead: Wheatsheaf

Denham Wright, J. and Pearl, L. (2000) 'The Experience and Knowledge of Young People Regarding Illicit Drug Use 1969–99'. *Addiction* 95(8): 1225–35

Department for Children, Schools and Families, Home Office and Department of Health (2008) *Youth Alcohol Action Plan*. London: The Stationery Office

Department for Children, Schools and Families (DCSF) (2010) *Working Together to Safeguard Children: A Guide to Inter-Agency Working to Safeguard and Promote the Welfare of Children*. www.education.gov.uk/publications/standard/publicationdetail/page1/dcsf-00305-2010, accessed 11 November 2013

Department of Education (2004) *Every Child Matters*. London: The Stationery Office

Department of Education (2012) *The Impact of SureStart Local Programmes on Seven-Year Olds and their Families*. DFE-RB220. www.ness.bbk.ac.uk/impact/documents/DFE-RB220.pdf

Department of Health (1996) *The Task Force to Review Services for Drug Misusers – Report of an Independent Review of Drug Treatment Services in England*. London: Department of Health

Department of Health (1998) *Health Action Zones*. Briefing paper distributed by the Central Drugs Prevention Unit, 19 May

Department of Health (1999) *Partnership in Action: New Opportunities for Joint Working between Health and Social Services*. www.doh.gov.uk/pia.htm

Department of Health (2002) *Mental Health Policy Implementation Guide: Dual Diagnosis Good Practice Guide*. London: Department of Health. www.nta.nhs.uk/uploads/prisons_dual_diagnosis_final_2009.pdf, accessed 5 September 2013

Department of Health (2011) *Public Health in Local Government*. www.dh.gov.uk/publications, accessed 1 April 2013

Department of Health (2012a) Health and Social Care Act. www.dh.gov.uk/publications, accessed 1 April 2013

Department of Health (2012b) Health and Social Care Fact Sheet. www.gov.uk/government/uploads/system/uploads/attachment_data/file/138257/A1.-Factsheet-Overview-240412.pdf, accessed 1 April 2013

Department of Health (2012c) *Smoking, Drinking and Drug Use among Young People in England in 2011*. A survey carried out for the Health and Social Care Information Centre NatCen Social Research and the National Foundation for Educational Research Health and Social Care Information Centre. www.ic.nhs.uk/webfiles/publications/003_Health_Lifestyles/smoking%20drinking%20drug%20use%202011/Smoking_drinking_and_drug_use_among_young_people_in_England_in_2011, accessed 19 November 2012

Department of Health (2012d) *UK Drug Situation: 2012 Edition*. UK Focal Point on Drugs Annual Report to the European Monitoring Centre on Drugs and Drug Addiction (EMCDDA) Centre for Public Health, Liverpool John Moores University, UK

Department of Health and Ministry of Justice (2009) *A Guide for the Management of Dual Diagnosis in Prisons* London: Department of Health

Der Spiegel (27 March 2013) 'This is Working: Portugal, 12 Years after Decriminalizing Drugs By Wiebke Hollersen'. www.spiegel.de/international/europe/evaluating-drug-decriminalization-in-portugal-12-years-later-a-891060.html, accessed 11 June 2013

Domosławski, A. (2011) 'Drug Policy in Portugal: The Benefits of Decriminalising Drug Use'. June. Open Society Foundations. www.opensocietyfoundations.org/sites/default/files/drug-policy-in-portugal-english-20120814.pdf, accessed 11 November 2013

Donnison, D. (1991) *A Radical Agenda: After the New Right and Old Left*. London: Oram Press

Downes, D. (1995) 'Crime and Inequality: Current Issues in Research and Public Debate Introduction'. Paper presented at the British Criminology Conference, 18–25 July

Druglink (January/February 1994) *Back to Basics Report Says Cut Drug Use to Curb HIV*. London: ISDD

Druglink (July/August 1997) *New Labour, New Broom*. London: ISDD

Drugs and Community Safety: The Strategic Challenge (10 December 1997) Report of a Local Government Drugs Forum Conference. London: HMSO

Drugs Prevention (1999) *Initiative: Final Progress Report 1997–1999*. London: Home Office Communication Directorate

DrugScope (13 October 2007) 'DrugScope "extremely disappointed" as calls for review of drug classification system ignored'. www.drugscope.org.uk/ourwork/pressoffice/pressreleases, accessed 18 November 2007

DrugScope (2013) 'Why do people die after taking ecstasy? The reasons and some statistics'. www.drugscope.org.uk/resources/faqs/faqpages/why-do-people-die-after-taking-ecstasy, accessed 3 September 2013

Duke, K. (2006) 'Out of Crime and into Treatment? The Criminalisation of Contemporary Drug Policy since *Tackling Drugs Together*'. *Drugs: Education, Prevention and Policy* 13(5): 409–15

Duke, K. and MacGregor, S. (1997) *Tackling Drugs Locally: The Implementation of DATs in England*. London: The Stationery Office

Duke, K., MacGregor, S. and Smith, L. (1995) *Activating Local Networks: A Comparison of Two Community Development Approaches to Drug Prevention*. London: The Stationery Office

Dunlap, E. (1995) 'Inner City Crisis and Drug Dealing:- Portrait of a New York Drug Dealer and His Household'. In S. MacGregor and A. Lipow (eds). *The Other City: People and Politics in New York and London*. Atlantic Highlands, NJ: Humanities Press

Edmunds, M., May, T., Hearnden, I. and Hough, M. (1998) *Arrest Referral: Emerging Lessons from Research*. DPI Paper 23. London: HMSO

Eisenstadt, N. (2011) 'Despite initial mistakes, the success of the Sure Start programme has been to prove that government does have a role to play in the development of young children'. 28 September. http://blogs.lse.ac.uk/politicsandpolicy/archives/15375, accessed 3 September 2013

Eisenstadt, N. (2013) 'Naomi Eisenstadt blog – Impressions of Early Years Strategy in Scotland 31st May 2013'. http://engageforeducation.org/2013/05/naomi-eisendtadt-blog-impressions-of-early-years-strategy-in-scotland/, accessed 5 September 2013

EMCDDA (2009) *Polydrug Use: Patterns and Responses*. Luxembourg: Publications Office of the European Union

EMCDDA (2011) *Drug Policy Profiles: Portugal, Luxembourg*. Luxembourg: Publications Office of the European Union

EMCDDA (2012a) *Annual Report 2012: The State of the Drugs Problem in Europe*. Luxembourg: Publications Office of the European Union

EMCDDA (2012b) *Children's Voices on Drug and Alcohol Use in Europe*. Luxembourg: Publications Office of the European Union

EMCDDA (2012c) *Country Overview: UK*. http://emcdda.europa.eu/publications/country-overview/uk, accessed 11 June 2013

Etzioni, A. (1993) *"The Spirit of Community: Rights, Responsibilities, and the Communitarian Agenda"*. New York: Crown Publishers

Etzioni, A. (1998) 'A Communitarian Note on Stakeholder Theory'. *Business Ethics Quarterly* 8(4): 679–91

European Commission (2013) *Further Insights into Aspects of the EU Illicit Drugs Market: Summaries and Findings*. Luxembourg: European Commission

Faggiano, F. Vigna-Taglianti, F.D., Versino, E., Zambon, A. Borraccino, A. and Lemma, P. (2005) 'School-Based Prevention for Illicit Drugs Use'. *Cochrane Database of Systematic Reviews*

Fakier, N. and Wild, L. (2011) 'Associations among Sleep Problems, Learning Difficulties and Substance Use in Adolescence'. *Journal of Adolescence* 34: 717–26

Farrall, S. and Hay, C. (2010) 'Not So Tough on Crime? Why Weren't the Thatcher Governments More Radical in Reforming the Criminal Justice System?' *British Journal of Criminology* 50(3): 550–69

Fast, D., Small, W., Krusl, A., Wood, E. and Kerr, T. (2012) '"I Guess my Own Fancy Screwed me Over": Transitions in Drug Use and the Context of Choice among Young People Entrenched in Open Drug Scene'. *BMC Public Health* 10: 126

Feeley, M.M and Simon, J. (1996) 'The New Penology' In J. Muncie, E. McLaughlin and M. Langan (eds), *Criminological Perspectives: A Reader*. London: Sage, 367–79

Field, F. (1996) *Stakeholder Welfare*. London: IEA Health and Welfare Unit

Fox, C. and Albertson, K. (2012) 'Is Payment by Results the Most Efficient Way to Address the Challenges Faced by the Criminal Justice Sector?' *Probation Journal* 59: 355–73

Fox, C.L., Towe, S.L., Stephens, R.S., Walker, D.D., and Roffman, R.A. (2011) 'Motives for Cannabis Use in High-Risk Adolescent Users'. *Psychology of Addictive Behaviours* 25(3): 492–500

Fox, D. and Arnull, E. (2013) *Social Work in the Youth Justice System: A Multidisciplinary Perspective*. Maidenhead: Open University Press

Fox News (4 June 2013) 'OAS Meeting Focuses on New Drug Strategies'. http://latino.foxnews.com/latino/news/2013/06/04/oas-meeting-focuses-on-new-drug-strategies/, accessed 9 June 2013

Foxcroft, D.R. and Tsertvadze, A. (2011) 'Universal School-Based Prevention Programs for Alcohol Misuse in Young People'. *Cochrane Database of Systematic Reviews*

Galvani, S. (2012) *Supporting People with Alcohol and Drug Problems: Making a Difference*. Bristol: Policy Press

Galvani, S. and Forrester, D. (2009) 'Social Work and Substance Use – Teaching the Basics'. SWAP. www.swap.ac.uk/docs/guide_su_learning&teaching.pdf

Galvani, S. and Hughes, N. (2010) 'Working with Alcohol and Drug Use: Exploring the Knowledge and Attitudes of Social Work Students'. *British Journal of Social Work* 40: 946–62

Galvani, S., Dance, C. and Hutchinson, A. (2011) 'From the Front Line: Alcohol, Drugs and Social Care Practice. A National Study'. Tilda Goldberg Centre, University of Bedfordshire

Geddes, M., Davies, J. and Fuller, C. (2007) 'Evaluating Local Strategic Partnerships: Theory and Practice of Change'. *Local Government Studies* 33(1): 97–116

Gelsthorpe, L. and Hedderman, C. (2012) 'Providing for Women Offenders: The Risks of Adopting a Payment by Results Approach'. *Probation Journal* 59(4): 374–90

Gilbert, R., Kemp, A., Thoburn, J., Sidebotham, P., Radford, L., Glaser, D. and MacMillan, H.L. (2009) 'Recognising and Responding to Child Maltreatment'. *The Lancet* 373: 167–80

Glendinning, C., Powell, M. and Rummery, K. (eds) (2002) *Partnerships, New Labour and the Governance of Welfare*. Bristol: Policy Press

Goodman, A. (2007) *Social Work with Drug and Substance Misusers*. Exeter: Learning Matters

Gossop, M., Marsden, J., Stewart, D. and Treacy, S. (2001) 'Outcomes after Methadone Maintenance and Methadone Reduction Treatments: Two-Year Follow-Up Results from the NTORS'. *Drugs and Alcohol Dependence* 62(3): 255–64

The Guardian (January 2013) 'Probation service leaders need support to implement reforms'. www.theguardian.com/society/2013/jan/22/probation-service-leaders-support-changes, accessed 2 September 2013

The Guardian (13 May 2013) 'Home Office tour to study drug policies in 10 countries'. www.guardian.co.uk/politics/2013/may/13/home-office-drug-policies-international, accessed 11 June 2013

The Guardian (16 May 2013) 'Users face growing threat from 200-plus synthetic drugs in circulation across UK, says government's chief drugs adviser'. www.guardian.co.uk/uk/2013/may/16/legal-highs-risk-overdose-drugs-tsar, accessed 9 June 2013

The Guardian (July 2013) 'Theresa May ignores experts and bans use of qat'. www.theguardian.com/politics/2013/jul/03/theresa-may-bans-qat, accessed 3 September 2013

Gudonis-Miller, L.C., Lewis, L. Tong, Y., Tu, W. and Aalsma, M. (2011) 'Adolescent Romantic Couples' Influence on Substance Use in Young Adulthood'. *Journal of Adolescence* 35: 638–47

Harris, C.C. (1989) 'The State and the Market'. In P. Brown and R. Sparks (eds), *Beyond Thatcherism: Social Policy, Politics and Society*. Milton Keynes: Open University Press, 1–16

Harwin, J., Ryan, M. and Tunnard, J. (2011) *The Family Drug and Alcohol Court Evaluation Report*. Brunel University, Nuffield Foundation and Coram

Hawthorne, G. (1996) 'The Social Impact of Life Education: Estimating Drug Use Prevalence among Victorian Primary School Students and the Statewide Effect of the Life Education Programme'. *Addiction* 91(8): 1151–60

Hay, G., Rael de Santos, G. and Millar, T. (2011) 'Estimate of the prevalence of opiate use and crack/cocaine use 2010/11: Sweep 7 report'. Centre for Public Health, Liverpool John Moores University

Hellawell, K. (2002) *The Outsider.* London: HarperCollins

Hickman, M., Sutcliffe, H., Sondhi, A. and Stimson, G.V. (1997) 'Validation of a Regional Drug Misuse Database: Implications for Policy and Surveillance of Problem Drug Use in the UK'. *British Medical Journal* 315: 581

Hill, M. and Hupe, P. (2006) 'Analysing Policy Processes as Multiple Governance: Accountability in Social Policy'. *Policy & Politics* 34(3): 557–73

Himmelstein, J.L. (1978) 'Drug Politics Theory: Analysis and Critique'. *Journal of Drug Issues* 8(1): 37–52

HM Government (1995) *Tackling Drugs Together: A Strategy for England 1995–1998* (Cmd 2846). London: HMSO

HM Government (1998) *Modern Public Services for Britain: Investing in Reform. Comprehensive Spending Review: New Public Spending Plans 1999–2002* (CM 4011). London: HMSO

HM Government (1998) *Tackling Drugs to Build a Better Britain: The Government's Ten-Year Strategy for Tackling Drugs Misuse* (Cmd 3945). London: HMSO

HM Government (1999) *Modernising Government* (Cmd 4310). London: HMSO

HM Government (2001) *Proceeds of Crime Bill: Publication of Draft Clauses* (CM 5066). London: HMSO

HM Government (2002) *Updated Drug Strategy.* London: HMSO

HM Government (2004) *Confident Communities in a Secure Britain: the Home Office Strategic Plan 2004–08* (CM 6287). London: HMSO

HM Government (2010) *Drug Strategy 2010: Reducing Demand, Restricting Supply, Building Recovery: Supporting People to Live a Drug Free Life.* London: Home Office

HM Government (2012) *Drug Strategy 2010: Reducing Demand, Restricting Supply, Building Recovery: Supporting People to Live a Drug Free Life. Annual Review – May.* London: Home Office

HM Government (2012) *The Government's Alcohol Strategy* (CM 8336). London: HMSO

HM Treasury (2000) *Cross-Departmental Review of Illegal Drugs.* www.archive.official-documents.co.uk/document/cm48/4807/chap29.html, accessed 30 September 2006

Home Affairs Committee (1986) *Misuse of Hard Drugs: Second Special Report from the Home Affairs Committee.* London: HMSO

Home Affairs Committee (2002) *The Government's Drug Strategy: Is It Working?* (HC 318). www.publications.parliament.uk/pa/cm200102/cmselect/cmhaff/318/31805, accessed 2 March 2004

Home Affairs Committee (2002) 'Report on drugs policy to be debated'. Press release 2002–03 no. 1. 29 November

Home Affairs Committee (2012) *Breaking the Cycle.* www.publications.parliament.uk/pa/cm201213/cmselect/cmhaff/184/18409.htm

Home Office (undated) *Let's Get Real: Communicating with the Public About Drugs.* London: HMSO

Home Office (1991) *Safer Communities: The Local Delivery of Crime Prevention through the Partnership Approach.* London: HMSO

Home Office (1997) *Tackling Drugs Together: Report of a Thematic Inspection on the Work of the Probation Service with Drug Misusers.* London: HMSO

Home Office (2001) *Making Punishments Work: Report of a Review of the Sentencing Framework for England and Wales.* London: HMSO

Home Office (2002) 'Educate, Prevent, and Treat – Key to Success in Tackling Drugs Problem: David Blunkett Publishes Updated Drug Strategy'. Press release

Home Office (2002) *Tackling Crack: A National Plan.* London: HMSO

Home Office (2003) *Home Office Departmental Report* (CM 5908). London: HMSO

Home Office (2007) *Drugs: Our Community, Your Say. A Consultation Paper.* London: HMSO

Home Office (2007) *Tackling Drugs: Changing Lives: Turning Strategy into Reality.* www.drugs.gov.uk

Home Office (2008) *Drugs: Protecting Families and Communities: The 2008 Drug Strategy.* London: HM Government

Hough, M. (1995) *Drugs Misuse and the Criminal Justice System: A Review of the Literature.* DPI Paper 15. London: HMSO

Howard, R. (2002) 'Are We on the Road to a Healthier Drugs Policy?' *Criminal Justice Matters* 47: 4–5

Howard, R., Beadle, P. and Maitland, J. (1993) *Across the Divide: Building Community Partnerships to Tackle Drug Misuse*. London: Department of Health

Hudson, B. and Hardy, B. (2002) 'What is a "Successful" Partnership and How Can it be Measured?' In C. Glendinning, M. Powell and K. Rummery (eds), *Partnerships, New Labour and the Governance of Welfare*. Bristol: Policy Press, 51–66

Huffington Post (6 April 2013) 'Latin America will push U.S. to discuss new drug war strategies at OAS Meeting'. www.huffingtonpost.com/2013/06/04/new-drug-war-strategy-_n_3383786.html, accessed 9 June 2013

Hunt, K., Sweeting, H., Sargent, J., Lewars, H., Young, R. and West, P. (2011) 'Is there an Association between Seeing Incidents of Alcohol or Drug Use in Films and Young Scottish Adults' Own Alcohol or Drug Use? A Cross Sectional Study'. *BMC Public Health* 11: 259

Hutchings, J., Bywater, T., Daley, D., Gardener, F., Whitaker, C., Jones, K., Eames, C. and Edwards, R.T. (2007) 'Parenting Intervention in Sure Start Services for Children at Risk of Developing Conduct Disorder: Pragmatic Randomised Controlled Trial'. *British Medical Journal* 334: 678

The Independent (8 January 2013) '"I don't want to die": Amy Winehouse's words just hours before her death'. www.independent.co.uk/arts-entertainment/music/news/i-dont-want-to-die-amy-winehouses-words-just-hours-before-her-death-8442698.html, accessed 4 September 2013

The Independent (1 February 2013) 'Chris Owen: my journey to sobriety'. www.independent.co.uk/voices/comment/alcoholics-anonymous-do-extraordinary-brave-work-for-people-who-are-in-need-but-my-journey-to-sobriety-shows-their-technique-isnt-for-everyone-8477252.html

Institute of Alcohol Studies (2010) *Binge Drinking – Nature, Prevalence and Causes*. St Ives, Cambs: IAS

International Federation of Social Workers (IFSW) (2012) 'Statement of Ethical Principles'. http://ifsw.org/policies/statement-of-ethical-principles/

Ives, R., Ghelani, P. and Mallick, J. (2004) 'Children, Young People and Health Related Decisions: The Implications for Health Education of Children and Young People'. Educari in association with Roehampton University

Jensen, C.D., Cushing, C.C., Aylward, B.S., Craig, J.T., Sorrell, D.M. and Steele, R.G. (2011) 'Effectiveness of Motivational Interviewing Interventions for Adolescent Substance Use Behaviour Change: A Meta-Analytic Review'. *Journal of Consulting and Clinical Psychology* 79(4): 433–40

Jepson, R.J., Harris, F.M., Platt, S. and Tannahill, C. (2010) 'The Effectiveness of Interventions to Change Six Health Behaviours: A Review of Reviews'. *BMC Public Health* 10: 538. http://biomedcentral.com

Joyce, R. and O'Connor, L. (2008) 'An Overview of the Underpinning Rationale and the Content, Delivery and Outcomes of Life Education Programmes'. *Life Education* (March)

JRF (2007) *Parenting and the Different Ways it can Affect Children's Lives: Research Evidence*. York: Joseph Rowntree Foundation

Kelly, J.F. and Hoeppner, B.B. (2013) 'Project MATCH: Rationale and Methods for a Multisite Clinical Trial Matching Patients to Alcoholism Treatment'. *Alcoholism: Clinical and Experimental Research* 17: 1130–45

Keys, D., Mallett, S. and Rosenthal, D. (2006) 'Giving up on Drugs: Homeless Young People and Self-Reported Drug Use'. *Contemporary Drug Problems* 33: 63–99

Kim, H.K. and Leve, L.D. (2011) 'Substance Use and Delinquency Among Middle School Girls in Foster Care: A Three-Year Follow-Up of a Randomized Controlled Trial'. *Journal of Consulting and Clinical Psychology* 79(6): 740–50

Klein, R. (1993) 'O'Goffe's Tale – or What Can We Learn from the Success of the Capitalist Welfare States?' In C. Jones (ed), *New Perspectives on the Welfare State in Europe Britain*. London: Routledge, 6–15

Lai, D.T.C., Cahill, K. and Tang, Q.Y. (2010) *Motivational Interviewing for Smoking Cessation*. New York: Cochrane Collaboration/John Wiley

Larsen, T.P., Taylor-Gooby, P. and Kananen, J. (2006) 'New Labour's Policy Style: A Mix of Policy Approaches'. *Journal of Social Policy* 35(4): 629–49

Leavey, G., Rothi, D. and Paul, R. (2011) 'Trust, Autonomy and Relationships: The Help-Seeking Preferences of Young People in Secondary Level Schools in London (UK)'. *Journal of Adolescence* 34: 685–93

Levin, P. (1997) *Making Social Policy: The Mechanisms of Government and Politics and How to Investigate Them*. Buckingham: Open University Press

Licensing Act (2003) www.gov.uk/alcohol-licensing, accessed 11 June 2011

Little, M. (2007) 'Sure Start made more credible by success of Incredible Years'. www.prevention.org./what-works/sure-start-made-more-credible-success-incredible-years/72, accessed 3 September 2013

Lowdnes, V. (2005) 'Something Old, Something New, Something Borrowed ...: How Institutions Change (and Stay the Same) in Local Governance'. *Policy Studies* 26(3/4): 291–309

MacGregor, S. (1998) 'Reluctant Partners: Trends in Approaches to Urban Drug-Taking in Contemporary Britain'. *Journal of Drug Issues* 28(1): 185–98

MacGregor, S. (1999) 'Medicine, Custom or Moral Fibre: Policy Responses to Drug Misuse'. In N. South (ed), *Drugs: Cultures, Controls and Everyday Life*. London: Sage, 67–85

MacGregor, S. (2006a) '*Tackling Drugs Together*: Ten Years On'. *Drugs: Education, Prevention and Policy* 13(5): 393–8

MacGregor, S. (2006b) '*Tackling Drugs Together* and the Establishment of the Principle that "Treatment Works"'. *Drugs: Education, Prevention and Policy* 13(5): 399–408

Macleod, J., Oakes, R., Copello, A., Crome, J., Egger, M., Hickman, M., Oppenkowski, T., Stokes-Lampard, H. and Davey Smith, G. (2004) 'Psychological and Social Sequelae of Cannabis and Other Illicit Drug Use by Young People: A Systematic Review of Longitudinal, General Population Studies'. *The Lancet* 365: 1579–88

Mallett, S., Rosenthal, D. and Keys, D. (2005) 'Young People, Drug Use and Family Conflict: Pathways into Homelessness'. *Journal of Adolescence* 28: 185–99

Marks, H. (2002) *The Howard Marks Book of Dope Stories*. London: Vintage

Marsden, J., Eastwood, B., Bradbury, C., Dale-Perera, A., Farrell, M., Hammond, P., Knight, J., Randhawa, K. and Wright, C. National Drug Treatment Monitoring System Outcomes Study Group (2009) 'Effectiveness of Community Treatments for Heroin and Crack Cocaine Addiction in England: A Prospective, In-Treatment Cohort Study'. *The Lancet* 10(374): 9697: 1262–70

Marsh, J.C. and Cao, D. (2005) 'Parents in Substance Abuse Treatment: Implications for Child Welfare Practice'. *Children and Youth Services Review* 27: 1259–78

Martino, S., Collins, R., Ellickson, P., Schell, T. and McCaffrey, D. (2006) 'Socio-Environmental Influences on Adolescents' Alcohol Outcome Expectancies: A Prospective Analysis', *Addiction* 101: 971–83

McAlaney, J. and McMahon, J. (2007) 'Diagnosing and Dealing with the "New British Disease"'. *The Psychologist* 20: 12738–41

McAlaney, J., Bewick, B. and Hughes, C. (2011) 'The International Development of the "Social Norms" Approach to Drug Education and Prevention'. *Drugs: Education, Prevention and Policy* 18(2): 81–9

McCrystal, P., Percy, A. and Higgins, K. (2007) 'The Cost of Drug Use in Adolescence: Young People, Money and Substance Use'. *Drugs: Education, Prevention and Policy* 14(1): 19–28

Measham, F. and Brain, K. (2005) '"Binge" Drinking, British Alcohol Policy and the New Culture of Intoxication'. *Crime, Media, Culture* 1(3): 262–83

Measham, F. and Moore, K. (2008) 'The Criminalisation of Intoxication'. In P. Squires (ed), *ASBO Nation: The Criminalisation of Nuisance*. Bristol: Policy Press, 273–88

Measham, F., Newcombe, R. and Parker, H. (1994) 'The Normalisation of Recreational Drug Use amongst Young People in North-West England'. *British Journal of Sociology* 45(2): 287–312

Measham, F., Parker, H. and Aldridge, J. (1998) *Starting, Switching, Slowing and Stopping: Report for the DPI Integrated Programme*. Paper 21. London: HMSO

Mid Staffordshire NHS Foundation Trust Public Inquiry (2013) *Report of the Mid Staffordshire NHS Foundation Trust Public Inquiry*. London: The Stationery Office

Miller, C.L., Pearce, M.E., Montinuzzamam, A., Thomas, V., Christian, W., Schecter, M.T. and Spittal, P.M. (2011) 'The Cedar Project: Risk Factors for Transition to Injecting Drug Use among Young Urban Aboriginal People'. *CMAJ* 183(10): 1147–54

Monk, R.L. and Heim, D. (2011) 'Self-Image Bias in Drug Use Attribution'. *Psychology of Addictive Behaviours* 25(4): 645–51

Moore, T.H.M., Zammit, S., Lingford-Hughes, A., Barnes, T.R.E., Jones, P.B., Burke, M. and Lewis, G. (2007) 'Cannabis Use and Risk of Psychotic or Affective Mental Health Outcomes: A Systematic Review'. *The Lancet* 370(9584): 319–28

Mott, J. (2000) 'Journal Interview 49: Conversation with Joy Mott'. *Addiction* 95(3): 329–37

Mounteney, J. (1996) 'DATs: How Have They Measured Up?' *Druglink* 11(4): 8–11

Mowlam, M. (2002) *Momentum: The Struggle for Peace, Politics and the People*. London: Hodder & Stoughton

Munro, E. (2011) *Munro on Child Protection: Final Report – A Child Centred System*. London: Department of Education. www.gov.uk/government/publications/munro-review-of-child-protection-final-report-a-child-centred-system, accessed 5 September 2013

Newman, J. (2001) *Modernising Governance: New Labour, Policy and Society*. London: Sage

NHS (2012) 'Smoking, drinking and drug use among young people in England in 2011'. Health and Social Care Centre

NSPCC (2009) *Teenagers at Risk: The Safeguarding Needs of Teenagers in Gangs and Violent Peer Groups*. London: NSPCC

NSPCC (July 2012) 'Gillick competency and Fraser guidelines'. Factsheet. www.nspcc.org.uk/inform/research/questions/gillick_wda61289.html, accessed 3 September 2013

NTA (2002). *Models of Care for the Treatment of Adult Drug Misusers*. London: NTA

NTA (2004). *Engaging and Retaining Clients in Drug Treatment*. London: NTA

NTA (2006) *Models of Care for Treatment of Adult Drug Misusers: Update 2006*. London: NTA

NTA (2007) *Assessing Young People for Substance Use*. London: NTA

NTA (2012) 'NTA prison drug treatment note for HAC 2012 drug policy review'. http://publications.parliament.uk/pa/cm201213/cmselect/cmhaff/184/184.09, accessed 21 July 2013

NTA (2013) *Chief Executive's Report to the Board March 2013*. NTA/Department of Health. www.nta.nhs.uk/uploads/paulsboardpaper.pdf, accessed 9 April 2013

NTA (2 April 2013) Drug and Alcohol Monitoring System (DAMS)

Nutt, D., King, L.A. and Phillips, L.D. (2010) 'Drug Harms in the UK: A Multicriteria Decision Analysis'. *The Lancet* 376: 1558–65

The Observer (5 May 2013) 'Inside Denmark's "fixing room", where nurses watch as addicts inject in safety'

Organisation of American States (OAS) (2013) *Report on the Drug Problem in the Americas: Terms of Reference*

Organisation for Economic Co-operation and Development (2010) *Improving Health and Social Cohesion through Education*. Paris: OECD

Parker, H. and Newcombe, R. (1987) 'Heroin Use and Acquisitive Crime in an English Community'. *British Journal of Sociology* 38(3): 331–50

Parker, H., Bury, C. and Egginton, R. (1998) *New Heroin Outbreaks amongst Young People in England and Wales*. Police Research Group: Crime Detection and Prevention Series Paper 92. London: Home Office

Parker, H., Williams, L. and Aldridge, J. (2002) 'The Normalisation of "Sensible" Recreational Drug Use: Further Evidence from the North West England Longitudinal Study'. *Sociology* 36(4): 941–64

Patel, S., Wright, S. and Gammampila, A. (2005) *Khat Use amongst Somalis in Four English Cities*. RDS 4705. London: Home Office

Paylor, I., Measham, F. and Asher, H. (2012) *Social Work and Drug Use*. Maidenhead: Open University Press

Pearson, G. (1987) *The New Heroin Users*. London: Blackwell

Pearson, G. (1991) 'Drug Control Policies in Britain'. *Crime and Justice* 14: 167–227

Perkins, H.W. and Berkowitz, A.D. (1986) 'Perceiving the Community Norms of Alcohol Use among Students: Some Research Implications for Campus Alcohol Education Programming'. *International Journal of the Addictions* 21: 961–76

Perra, O., Fletcher, A., Bonell, C., Higgins, K. and McCrystal, P. (2012) 'School Related Predictors of Smoking, Drinking and Drug Use: Evidence from the Belfast Youth Development Study'. *Journal of Adolescence* 35: 315–24

Poulin, F., Kiesner, J., Pedersen, S. and Dishion, T.J. (2011) 'A Short-Term Longitudinal Analysis of Friendship Selection on Early Adolescent Substance Use'. *Journal of Adolescence* 34: 249–56

Powell, M. and Dowling, B. (2006) 'New Labour's Partnerships: Comparing Conceptual Models with Existing Forms'. *Social Policy and Society* 5(2): 305–14

Powell, M. and Exworthy, M. (2002) 'Partnerships, Quasi-Networks and Social Policy'. In C. Glendinning, M. Powell and K. Rummery (eds), *Partnerships, New Labour and the Governance of Welfare*. Bristol: Policy Press, 15–32

Prison Reform Trust (2010) 'The Prison Reform Trust response to the NHS White Paper, *Equity and Excellence*: Liberating the NHS'. London: Prison Reform Trust

Prochaska, J. and diClemente, C.C. (1982) 'Transtheoretical Therapy: Towards a More Integrative Model of Change'. *Psychotherapy: Theory, Research & Practice* 19(3): 276–88

Prochaska, J. and diClemente, C.C. (1998) 'Towards a Comprehensive Transtheoretical Model of Change: Stages of Change and Addictive Behaviours'. In W.R. Miller and N. Heather (eds), *Treating Addictive Behaviors*, 2nd edn. New York: Plenum Press, 3–24

Reuter, P. and Stevens, A. (2007) *An Analysis of UK Drug Policy*. London: UKDPC

Rosenkranz, S.E., Muller, R.T. and Henderson, J.L. (2012) 'Psychological Maltreatment in Relation to Substance Use Problem Severity among Youth'. *Child Abuse and Neglect* 36: 438–48

Rummery, K. (2006) 'Partnerships and Collaborative Governance in Welfare: The Citizenship Challenge'. *Social Policy and Society* 5:(2): 293–303

Sackett, D.L., Rosenberg, W.M.C., Muir Gray, J.A., Haynes, R.B. and Richardson, W.S. (1996) 'Evidence Based Medicine: What It Is and What It Isn't'. *British Medical Journal* 312: 71–2

Saenz de Ugarte, L. and Martin-Aranaga, I. (2012) 'Social Work and Risk Society: The Need for Shared Social Responsibility'. *European Journal of Social Work* 14(4): 447–62

Sanderson, I. (2006) 'Complexity, "Practical Rationality" and Evidence-Based Policy Making'. *Policy & Politics* 34(1): 11–32

Seddon, T. (2006) 'Drugs, Crime and Social Exclusion'. *British Journal of Criminology* 46: 680–703

Seddon, T., Williams, L. and Ralphs, R. (2012) *Tough Choices*. Clarendon Studies in Criminology. Oxford: Oxford University Press

Shiner, M. and Newburn, T. (1999) 'Taking Tea with Noel: The Place and Meaning of Drug Use in Everyday Life'. In N. South (ed), *Drugs: Cultures, Controls and Everyday Life*. London: Sage, 139–59

Sixty-Seventh General Assembly Plenary 3rd, 4th & 5th Meetings (AM, PM & Night) (24 September 2012) 'World leaders adopt declaration reaffirming rule of law as foundation for building equitable state relations, just societies'. www.un.org/News/Press/docs/2012/ga11290.doc.htm, accessed 3 September 2013

Smith, D., McVie, S., Woodward, R., Shute, J., Flint, J. and McAra, L. (2001) *The Edinburgh Study of Youth Transitions and Crime: Key Findings at Ages 12 and 13*. www.law.ed.ac.uk/cls/esytc/findingsreport.htm

Society of Editors and UKDPC (2012) *Dealing with the Stigma of Drugs: Guidance for Journalists*. Cambridge: Society of Editors

South, N. (1999) 'Debating Drugs and Everyday Life: Normalisation, Prohibition and "Otherness"'. In N. South (ed), *Drugs: Cultures, Controls and Everyday Life*. London: Sage, 1–16

Steinhagen, K.A. and Freidman, M.B (2008) 'Substance Abuse and Misuse in Older Adults'. *Aging Well* 3(20). http://todaysgeriatricmedicine.com/archive/071708p20.shtml, accessed 5 September 2013

Stimson, G.V. (1987) 'British Drug Policies in the 1980s: A Preliminary Analysis and Suggestions for Research'. *British Journal of Addiction* 82(5): 477–88

Stimson, G.V. (2000) 'Hard Labour: Blair Welfare'. *Druglink* 15(4): 10–12

Strang, J. (2012) *Medications in Recovery: Reorienting Drug Dependence Treatment*. London: NTA

Strengthening the Evidence Base for the UK Drugs Strategy: A Consultation Event (2004) Home Office RDS Conference

The Sunday Times (21 April 2013) 'Comment: Get Brighton to A&E – it's overdosing on liberal claptrap'. www.thesundaytimes.co.uk/sto/comment/columns/rodliddle/article1248291.ece, accessed 11 November 2013

The Sunday Times (25 August 2013) 'Beaten, raped, starved: the teenage ghosts behind the cannabis trade'. www.thesundaytimes.co.uk/sto/news/focus/article1304823.ece, accessed 11 November 2013

Taylor, M. (2001) 'Partnership: Insiders and Outsiders'. In M. Harris and C. Rochester (eds), *Voluntary Organisations and Social Policy in Britain*. Basingstoke: Palgrave Macmillan, 94–107

Thom, B. (1999) *Dealing with Drink: Alcohol and Social Policy – From Treatment to Management*. London: Free Association Books

Thompson, N. (2001) *Anti-Discriminatory Practice*, 3rd edition. Basingstoke: Palgrave Macmillan

Towe, N. (undated) 'Comment on TDTBBB'. Unpublished paper for Local Government Association

Townsend P. (1993) 'Underclass and Overclass: The Widening Gulf Between Social Classes in Britain in the 1980s'. In M. Cross and G. Payne (eds), *Sociology in Action*. Basingstoke: Macmillan, 91–118

Trace, M. (2003) 'Snakes and Ladders: Five Years Inside Government Drug Policy'. *Druglink* (March/April): 8–9

Transform (22 July 2013) 'Help make legal cannabis a reality'. http://transform-drugs.blogspot.co.uk/2013/07/help-make-legal-cannabis-reality.html, accessed 3 September 2013

Trautmann, F., Kilmer, B. and Turnbull, P. (2013) *Further Insights into Aspects of the EU Illicit Drugs Market: Summaries and Key Findings*. European Commission – Directorate-General for Justice. Luxembourg: Publications Office for the European Union

Turnball, P., Webster, R. and Stillwell, G. (1995) *Get it While You Can: An Evaluation of an Early Intervention Project for Arrestees with Alcohol and Drug Problems*. DPI Series Paper 9. London: HMSO

Turning Point (2007) *Dual Diagnosis Good Practice Handbook*. London: Turning Point

Tyler, A. (1986) *Street Drugs: The Facts Explained, the Myths Exploded*, 2nd edition 1995. London: Hodder & Stoughton

UK Drug Policy Commission (UKDPC) (2007) 'Response to the UK Government's Drug Strategy Consultation Paper October 2007'. www.ukdpc.org.uk/reports, accessed 18 November 2007

UK Drug Policy Commission (UKDPC) (2010) *The Problem with Stigma: The Problem with Stigmatising Drug Users*. London: NTA

UK Drug Policy Commission (UKDPC) (2012) *A Fresh Approach to Drugs: The Final Report of the UK Drug Policy Commission*. www.ukdpc.org.uk/reports, accessed 30 October 2012

University of Stirling News (1 August 2013) 'Government under pressure as Australian study shows support for plain-packaged cigarettes'. www.stir.ac.uk/news/news-archive/13/08/support-for-plain-packs-bmj/, accessed 4 September 2013

van Amsterdam, J.G.C., Opperhuizen, A., Koeter, M. and van den Brink, W. (2010) 'Ranking the Harm of Alcohol, Tobacco and Illicit Drugs for the Individual and the Population'. *European Addict Research* 16: 202–27

van Oorschot, W. (2000) 'Who Should Get What and Why? On Deservingness Criteria and the Conditionality of Solidarity among the Public'. *Policy & Politics* 28(1): 33–48

Vanwormer, K., Vanwormer, R. and Dickenson, S. (1999) 'Regarding Heroin: British and American Approaches'. *International Journal of Social Work* 42(3): 319–31

Velleman, R. and Orford, J. (eds) (1999) *Risk and Resilience: Adults Who Were the Children of Problem Drinkers*. London: Harwood Academic

Vuillamy, E. (24 July 2011). 'Richard Nixon's "war on drugs" began 40 years ago, and the battle is still raging'. *The Guardian*

Wales, G.A., Hill, L. and Robertson, F. (2009) *Untold Damage: Children Living with Parents Who Drink Harmfully*. Glasgow: ChildLine Scotland/SHAAP

Wallace, S.K and Staiger, P.K. (1998) 'Informing Consent: Should "Providers" Inform "Purchasers" About the Risks of Drug Education?' *Health Promotion International*. http://heapro.oxfordjournals.org/content/13/2/167.short, accessed 5 September 2013

Wanigarante, S., Davies, P., Price, K. and Brotchie, J. (2005) 'The Effectiveness of Psychological Therapies on Drug Misusing Clients'. Research Briefings 11. London: NTA

Webber, R. (2002) 'Vietnamese-Australian Young People and Illicit Drug Use in Melbourne: Generation Gaps and Fault Lines'. *Youth Studies Australia* 21(3): 17–24

Whitehead, M. (2007) 'The Architecture of Partnerships: Urban Communities in the Shadow of Hierarchy', *Policy & Politics* 35(1): 3–23

Williams, T. (1998) *Making it Happen: An Evaluation of the DPI's Contribution to Local Partnerships*. London: The Stationery Office

Wilson, D., Croxson, B. and Atkinson, A. (2006) '"What Gets Measured Gets Done": Headteachers' Responses to the English Secondary School Performance Management System'. *Policy Studies* 27(2): 153–71

Wilson, H., Bryant, J., Holt, M. and Treloar, C. (2010) 'Normalisation of Recreational Drug Use among Young People: Evidence about Accessibility, Use and Contact with Drug Users'. *Health Sociology Review* 19(2): 164–75

Withington, P. (2013) Talk on '"Addictions": An Early Modern Perspective' on the *Addiction: Myth and Reality* panel as part of the British Library 'Myth and Reality' Series, 18 March

Woman's Own (23 September 1987) Douglas Keay, Margaret Thatcher and 'No such Thing as Society'. Also available at http://en.wikiquote.org/wiki/Margaret_Thatcher, accessed 7 June 2013 and Pro Thatcher – The Commentator –

'no such thing as society', Ghaffar Hussain at www.thecommentator.com/article/3276/no_such_thing_as_society, accessed 7 June 2013

Wong, C. (1998) 'Interrelationships between Key Actors in Local Economic Development'. *Environment and Planning C: Government and Policy* 16(4): 463–81

Yates, R. (2002) 'A Brief History of British Drug Policy 1950–2001'. *Drugs: Education, Prevention and Policy* 19(2): 113–24

Young, R. and West, P. (2010) 'Do "Good Values" Lead to "Good" Health Behaviours? Longitudinal Associations between Young People's Values and Later Substance-Use'. *BMC Public Health* 10: 165

Index